More Praise for *Women Rowing North*

"[Pipher's] 'quest for joy and happiness' is sincere, as is her commitment to helping other women achieve theirs . . . All readers will admire her unadorned but wise summation that answered prayers are 'a surcease of worry.'" —*The Washington Post*

"Thoughtful, wise, and profoundly transformative. This is truly a one of a kind book." —Julia Alvarez, author of *How the García Girls Lost Their Accents* and *Once Upon a Quinceañera*

"[A] wisdom-filled guide . . . Pipher's mindful tips act as a map to joy and remind us that we can flourish through *all* of our years." —*Woman's World*

"An illuminating, much-needed template for moving through advancing years with gratitude and grace." —Barbara Graham, *New York Times* bestselling author and editor of *Eye of My Heart*

"Sets the direction, shows the dangers, and brings the reader safely through to joy. I feel gratitude, not only for life, but for this wonderful book." —Jane Isay, author of *Unconditional Love*

"A work chock-full of wisdom and consoling messages." —*Publishers Weekly* (starred review)

"Simultaneously honest and calming. A profound and comforting guide to living deftly and deeply well into old age." —Meg Cox, author of *The Book of New Family Traditions*

"[Pipher] writes with authority and authenticity, shaping her accumulated wisdom with her artful writer's voice . . . The book is a gift that provides comfort, caring, and a positive way forward." —*More Content Now*

"This positive, affirming book will inspire and guide women facing these challenges." —*Booklist*

"Written with eloquence and commitment. The women [Pipher] describes have earned the right to be both present and accounted for." —Robert Fulford, *National Post*

"I love this book. Don't stop with a once-through reading. I myself keep it at hand to dip into for a quick shot of Mary Pipher's matter-of-fact wisdom, humor, and instinct for the essential. It never fails." —Joanna Macy, author of *Coming Back to Life*

WOMEN ROWING NORTH

Navigating Life's Currents
and Flourishing As We Age

MARY PIPHER

BLOOMSBURY PUBLISHING

NEW YORK · LONDON · OXFORD · NEW DELHI · SYDNEY

To all the women who have traveled with me along the river

BLOOMSBURY PUBLISHING
Bloomsbury Publishing Inc.
1385 Broadway, New York, NY 10018, USA

BLOOMSBURY, BLOOMSBURY PUBLISHING, and the Diana logo
are trademarks of Bloomsbury Publishing Plc

First published in the United States 2019
This paperback edition published 2020

Barbara Crooker, excerpt from "Equinox" on page 53 from *Barbara Crooker: Selected Poems*, copyright © 2015. Edna St. Vincent Millay, excerpt from "Dirge Without Music" on page 69 from *Collected Poems*. Copyright 1928, © 1955 by Edna St. Vincent Millay and Norma Millay Ellis. Reprinted with the permission of The Permissions Company, Inc., on behalf of Holly Peppe, Literary Executor, The Millay Society, www.millay.org. "Our True Heritage" on page 171 reprinted from *Call Me By My True Names* (1999) by Thich Nhat Hanh with permission of Parallax Press, Berkeley, California, www.parallax.org.

Bloomsbury Publishing Plc does not have any control over, or responsibility for, any third-party websites referred to or in this book. All internet addresses given in this book were correct at the time of going to press. The author and publisher regret any inconvenience caused if addresses have changed or sites have ceased to exist, but can accept no responsibility for any such changes.

ISBN: HB: 978-1-63286-960-9; PB: 978-1-63286-961-6; eBook: 978-1-63286-962-3

Library of Congress Cataloging-in-Publication Data is available.

2 4 6 8 10 9 7 5 3 1

Typeset by Westchester Publishing Services
Designed by Elizabeth Van Itallie
Printed and bound in the U.S.A. by Berryville Graphics Inc., Berryville, Virginia

To find out more about our authors and books visit www.bloomsbury.com
and sign up for our newsletters.

Bloomsbury books may be purchased for business or promotional use.
For information on bulk purchases please contact Macmillan Corporate
and Premium Sales Department at specialmarkets@macmillan.com.

Contents

Foreword

Since the publication of *Women Rowing North* in January of 2019, I have been deeply touched by the many letters I received. Women have written to tell me of their struggles with aging, including loss of vision, troubles with adult children, or fears of falling and breaking bones. Many women felt my book helped them build better days and develop more resilient personalities. Some said that the book had given them hope when they had been expecting to live in despair the rest of their lives. One woman wrote that, after two broken hips and her husband's death, she had given up, but that *Women Rowing North* showed her a path forward.

Other women wrote to say they were already strong copers and skillful at happiness. They were proud someone was telling their story. Some sent pictures of their kayaks, their gardens, or themselves with their friends on campouts. After reading about my hand pain and many hand surgeries, some women offered me advice. One woman gave me a Celtic hand meditation that I found healing. The readers' trust and kindness made me cry.

A few raised topics for further exploration. I heard from "elder orphans" who were aging and fearful there would be no one to help them as they aged. Widowed and divorced women wanted to know about dating in their sixties and seventies. Others asked for more examples of women caring for family members with chronic, debilitating illnesses.

Even men have written to say that they liked the book and felt it applied to them. (Several joked that I should write a new volume called *Men Going South*.) Many book clubs selected *Women Rowing North*, and several medical centers and universities built curriculums around its ideas. I have enjoyed thinking of women drinking wine or tea and discussing the book's themes, such as creating transcendent narratives or the power of yes and the power of no. I am pleased that teaching centers found the ideas in my book worthy of promulgating. These centers were also looking for better cultural education about aging and identity. People cannot change unless they have a vision of the change that is possible. I tried to offer that vision.

All these responses indicate that the book's timing was spot on. It turns out that my generation of women wants a fresh paradigm for aging. Our lives are not like our mothers' lives and we are weary of ageist, sexist portrayals of older women. The letters also validated my own informed optimism about the nature of humans. Almost all of us want to grow to our full potential and to be the happiest, most useful and loving people we can possibly be. We are eager to learn how to live deeper, more authentic lives.

As a baby boomer myself, I was eager to frame issues around older women in more positive and growth-enhancing ways. In *Women Rowing North*, I share all I know about being happy and leading a meaningful life rich in relationships.

Of course, I keep discovering new stories. For example, one of my friends who moved into a care facility was able to convince the facility's owner to let her supervise the growing of fresh vegetables for the residents. When I visited Kay in March, the halls around her room were filled with organic plants and grow lights. Kay could water these plants from her wheelchair. By July, when we toured the outdoor garden, she was providing kale, lettuce, carrots, and green beans to the kitchen. Fresh corn was on the way. When Kay told me how much the residents liked homegrown tomatoes, she beamed with pride and pleasure.

Since I wrote *Women Rowing North*, I have officiated at a funeral of a friend's husband and helped her grieve the loss of her partner of fifty years and adjust to a new life. I've walked with her on icy trails around

Holmes Lake at sunset and just lately I've danced with her at outdoor summer events where my husband's band provided the music. I have seen how a community of kind people gather around the grieving and help them live on with hope and a sense of belonging.

This is one of the great things about life. Every day beautiful new stories fall around us like light.

I hope all of you new readers find *Women Rowing North* useful. I continue to be grateful for the gift of life and am honored to share my time and place with so many wonderful people. I truly wish all of you the best on your journeys north.

Women Rowing North

Navigating Life's Currents and Flourishing as We Age

"I have everything I need to be happy right between my ears."
—Jane Jarvis

WOMEN ROWING NORTH is about the specific issues women face as we transition from middle age to old age. The core concern of this life stage, with all of its perils and pleasures, is how to cultivate resilient responses to the challenges we face. Resilience is built by attention and intention. We can take responsibility for our attitudes and focus on our strengths and our joys. We can go deep and face truth squarely. We can learn the skills that allow us to adapt to anything. Yes, anything.

With each new stage of life, we outgrow the strategies that worked for us at an earlier stage. We find ourselves in an environment that pelts us with more challenges than our current self can manage. If we don't grow bigger, we can become bitter. When our problems become too big for us, our healthiest response is to expand our capacities. That growth is qualitative. We become deeper, kinder to ourselves and others, and more capable of bliss.

Attitude is not everything, but it is almost everything. In fact, in many situations, it is all we have. Especially as we age, we can see clearly that we do not always have control, but we do have choices. That is our power. These choices determine whether we stagnate or grow into fully realized people.

Of course, the world is not divided into two types of women: those who grow and those who don't. All of us fit into both groups almost every day of our lives. Some of the time, we are good copers and resilient human beings; in other moments, we are reactive and pessimistic. Pain, sorrow, and anger will always be with us. But with will, intentionality, and the right set of skills, we can be happier over the long haul.

There are some lucky people who seem to be naturally sunny, but for many of us, happiness doesn't come easily. My knowledge about happiness comes from being someone who has struggled with sadness and anxiety much of my life.

I know how to take care of others and to be good, but it has been a lifelong journey to learn to take care of myself. I am from a family tree whose fruits include psychosis, depression, alcoholism, and suicide. As a girl I suffered a great deal of parental absence and I became the overly responsible, hyper-vigilant big sister. Once I told a friend I was theoretically happy and she laughed. She said, "You can't be theoretically happy any more than you can be theoretically orgasmic."

Even though I would not call my quest for joy and happiness a rousing success, I have learned from my journey. I don't expect constant happiness. Now, when I am blue, I know how to help myself. I am calmer and less reactive. I still have my share of bad days and I need constant reminders to be present and grateful, but I am engaged in a hopeful process. The process, rather than a perfect outcome, is what makes me happy.

To be happy at this junction, we cannot just settle for being a diminished version of our younger selves. We must change the ways we think and behave. This book focuses on the attitudes and skills we need in order to let go of the past, embrace the new, cope with loss, and experience wisdom, authenticity, and bliss.

During this life stage, we lose some of the long-term aspects of our identity, but we add new aspects and expand on many others. We learn to balance the loss of certain roles with the crafting of fresh and more serviceable ones. Hopefully, we become more gentle and kind to ourselves.

My focus is on women who, like myself, are on the cusp of change. I turn seventy this year. Women in their sixties and early seventies are crossing a border and everything interesting happens at borders.

Of course, women may feel that they are on this border at different ages. Chronological age is not as important as health. In the twenty-first century, we women often consider ourselves middle-aged well into our sixties. Until we suffer a major health crisis or the loss of someone we love, we continue to feel young.

Developmental psychologist Bernice Neugarten made this distinction between young-old age and old-old age. As long as we can do most of what we want to do, we are young-old age. When our health fundamentally changes the way we live, we have entered old-old age. However, my own experience is that many of us are between those two categories with various kinds of health problems, such as failing eyesight or arthritis. We still live much as we always have, but with adaptations.

Anthropologist Mary Catherine Bateson documents the extended life span of people born after World War II. Most of us have the possibility of living well into our eighties or nineties. She suggests that we call these later decades Adulthood II.

Throughout this book, I draw on my own experience. I've been a daughter, a big sister, a wife, a mother, a grandmother, and a caregiver for my ill sister with dementia. I've watched my parents die and held all five of my grandchildren on the first day of their lives.

I've been a therapist who worked primarily with women. My research has been on women. I taught Psychology of Women and Sex Roles and Gender at the University of Nebraska and I have written and spoken about women all of my professional life.

I write as a cultural anthropologist and clinical psychologist who specializes in developmental psychology and trauma. In *Reviving Ophelia: Saving the Selves of Adolescent Girls*, published in 1994, I wrote about teenagers; in *Women Rowing North*, I reflect on older women. Both life stages are sharp turns in the river requiring us to expand our identities.

As with *Reviving Ophelia*, this book explores a specific life stage from a feminist perspective, revealing the reality of women's lives as opposed to the dominant cultural stories about us. We are much more complicated, intense, and fascinating than most of America's stories suggest.

Our culture presents us with a misogynistic version of who we older women are. We confront both ageism and gender-specific challenges. As we age, our bodies, our sexuality, and our minds are devalued. There are many negative stereotypes about older women, but my least favorites manifest as mother-in-law jokes. These jokes suggest we are nosy, bossy, judgmental, and in the way. *Women Rowing North* begins a new conversation about our complexity, challenges, and gifts.

Contrary to cultural stereotypes, many older women are deeply happy. A 2014 Brookings Institute study on happiness and age found that people are least happy in their twenties, thirties, and early forties, and steadily gain an appreciation for life as they age. Indeed, most women become increasingly happy after age fifty-five, with their peak of happiness toward the very end of life.

Dilip Jeste at the University of California, San Diego, found in 2016 that as people age they report higher levels of overall satisfaction, happiness, and well-being, and lower levels of anxiety, depression, and stress. The older the person, the better her mental health tended to be. Women's happiness ratings were consistently higher than those of men. Recent census data from the United Kingdom finds that the happiest people are women aged 65–79.

There are many theories about why women fare better than men. One is simply that we tend to be healthier and more active. We also are more likely to have close relationships with family and friends. We understand how to hold intimate conversations, talk about our own deepest emotions, and help others discuss theirs. We may have a long-term partner and often have decades-old friendships to support us.

This year I experienced a vivid illustration of the happiness of older women. I switched recreational centers from the university where I have taught for many years to a gym geared toward older people. I noticed a great change in the locker room atmosphere. At the university, the young women were mostly stressed and unhappy. They talked on their phones or to their exercise partners about their weight, finances, studies, and relationship issues. Almost all of them hid their bodies by crouching as they undressed. Except for occasional happy talk about weekends or school holidays, conversation was generally gloomy.

On the other hand, in my new locker room, we older women walk around unselfconsciously naked or in utilitarian underclothes or swimsuits. Our bodies are saggy with plenty of stretch marks, wrinkles, and cellulite, but do we care? Not much.

We are more interested in each other's faces, which reveal decades of joy and suffering and are often open and awake to the moment.

Older women do talk about their troubles, especially what we call the "organ recitals," that is, conversations about health issues. Mostly, though, we discuss family, travel, books, movies, and fun. We joke around. For example, one day I heard a woman say, "The kinder you are to them the longer they last." Another woman asked, "What are you referring to?" Then, one by one, the rest of us chimed in, "Your knees," "Your bank account," "Your swimsuit," and "Your husband."

How do we manage our many difficulties? In this book, I argue that neither our genetics nor our external circumstances determine our happiness. Rather, happiness depends on how we deal with what we are given.

Even though we all suffer, we don't all grow. Not all older women become elders. Successful resolutions of our developmental challenges don't just happen. We don't become our wisest selves without effort. Our growth requires us to become skilled in perspective taking, in managing our emotions, in crafting positive narratives, and in forming intimate relationships. We develop the skills of building joy, gratitude, and meaning into every day. By learning these lessons, we cultivate emotional resilience.

We have the capacity to build happiness into our lives with humor, concern for others, and gratitude. Of course, we can't do it all of the time. That self-expectation would drive us crazy. However, we can develop habits that make it more likely that we will respond in an upbeat manner.

It's critical to distinguish between choosing to live lovingly and cheerfully and living a life of denial. One leads to joy, the other to emotional death. I have learned from my work as a therapist that secrets, denial, and avoidance invariably cause trouble. To move forward requires seeing clearly.

When we lose a beloved or learn that our health is deteriorating, our natural response is full-body despair. We are likely to panic, go numb, and wonder if we can survive. As we emerge from shock, we feel all the other painful emotions as well. We don't heal without hurting. For a while, the cure for the pain is the pain.

I don't recommend controlling our emotions, but rather listening to them. They are delivering information that is vital to our recovery. We want to fully experience our emotions in both our hearts and our bodies. If we do this, we will gradually move toward healing and hope.

Part of what allows us to deeply appreciate our lives and savor our time is our past despair. In fact, it has great value as a springboard for growth. There is an ancient and almost universal cycle that involves trauma, despair, struggle, adaptation, and resolution. This is a deepening cycle that prepares us for whatever comes next. It opens our hearts to others and helps us feel grateful for every small pleasure.

My role models are not women who avoided reality, but rather social activists such as Alice Paul, Tillie Olsen, and Grace Boggs who saw reality clearly and set about to improve it. I have always admired the multifaceted genius Margaret Fuller. In the early 1800s, she campaigned for birth control and women's rights. She once declared, "I accept the universe." She accepted it, in that she understood it and didn't deny reality, but she acted both to benefit women and to enjoy her life to the fullest.

Let us all reach for the freedom to see, hear, and feel everything. That does not mean we act on impulse. Rather, it means that, like Margaret Fuller, we have the fortitude to face the truth directly and then build our happiness accordingly.

Our journey through this life stage, while potentially beautiful, is arduous. Old age is always accompanied by loss. Eventually, one way or another, we will say goodbye to everyone we love. In our sixties and seventies, we are likely to spend more time in doctor's offices than at concerts and more time at funerals than weddings. Maneuvering this stretch of river requires flexibility, a tolerance for ambiguity, openness to new vistas, and the ability to conceptualize all experiences in positive ways.

Older women have the most need for navigational skills, but we also have the most experience acquiring them. We have weathered strong storms and hold a long view of life's journey. We can take responsibility for the emotional weather we create and experience.

This developmental stage is a "both/and" experience. Most likely, we will feel both some of life's deepest sorrows and also enjoy moments of bliss. Around the time of a parent's death, we may hold our first grandchild in our arms. We may have health issues that limit our mobility, but we can still savor a Bach concerto, bake a peach pie for a daughter's visit, or pack a picnic and watch the sunset from a beach or prairie.

If we make good choices and develop the skills discussed in this book, we will experience growth spurts. Let's aim to become more curious and less worried and more self-aware and less reactive. We can learn to embrace everything. All of it. Regardless of life circumstances and our innate human foibles, we can find serenity, happiness, and wisdom.

Women Rowing North is a guidebook for the flourishing that is possible. It explores what sustains, enlivens, and enriches us as we navigate this developmental stage. This era offers us an opportunity for emotional, social, and spiritual development. Perhaps the book's core lesson is simply "Everything is workable." We can always find the silver current of resilience that can carry us forward.

This book is both descriptive and prescriptive. I share what I learned about growth from my lifelong work as a therapist. I describe through interviews and stories the myriad points of view of women in this developmental stage. We learn from each other. This is not a "how to" book, but what I hope is a "how to think" book.

I interviewed women from all over the country and from many different educational, economic, and cultural backgrounds. I do not identify women by race, but Latina, Asian, Caucasian, African American, and Native American women all shared their stories. These women varied greatly in both what they were coping with and how well they were managing to cope. Some were in the depths of sorrow. Others were skilled in the art of vibrant living. But all were striving to master the challenges of this life stage. They were trying their best to be both happy and good.

Except for a few women who asked that I use their real names, the women I interviewed are given new names. Some stories are combined and details are changed to protect anonymity. I tell the stories of many women in this book; however, I focus on four women across time—Willow, Kestrel, Emma, and Sylvia.

I include many of my own stories and reflections. I know myself better than I can ever know anyone else. I see myself as a typical older woman. I'm middle-class and live in the middle of the country in a midsize university town. It's a blue city in a bright red state. I am mostly healthy, but I've lost some functioning. I am full of moods, flaws, disappointments, and self-criticism, and I will be trying to improve myself on my deathbed.

Women our age vary by race, cultural background, employment, socioeconomic status, geographic region, and sexual preferences. Likewise, we range from women who are full-time caregivers to those who have no such responsibilities. We differ in our access to resources, such as nearby family, life partners, close women friends, and safe and connected communities. I know women who are sixty going on ninety, while others, like my seventy-five-year-old friend Debbie from Los Angeles, are ready for yet another great adventure. We vary in the amount of emotional and physical pain we are suffering and in the amount of resilience we can summon. Some women seem hard to lift up and others are impossible to keep down.

Most of us exist between those extremes. We are resilient on some days but not others. We recover quickly from one kind of stress, but struggle to bounce back after another. What we share is our place on the river.

There is no one woman who can represent all of us. We are partnered and single, healthy and infirm, and contented and miserable. Thirty percent of women between sixty-five and sixty-nine are working. This book merely samples the richness and variety of women in our life stage.

Part I of *Women Rowing North* considers the challenges of aging, including ageism and lookism, caregiving, loss, and loneliness. Part II considers the travel skills necessary for our river journey north. These include understanding ourselves, skillful choices, community building, managing our narratives, and gratitude. I emphasize the importance of being useful. Barbara Kingsolver said it best: "Happy people have found a use for themselves like a good tool." Part III turns readers toward the lifeboat of long-term loving relationships. Whether or not we have a family, we need to live interdependently with others. Our growth depends on interaction: isolation is the quickest path to stagnation. Finally, Part IV explores the rewards of this life stage, including authenticity, enhanced perspectives, and bliss.

For this book's title I chose the word "rowing" rather than sailing or floating because, to stay on course, we need to make an effort, choose a positive attitude, and maintain a strong sense of direction as we travel toward winter and the land of snow and ice.

I feel fortunate to have a community of women friends who have gathered for thirty years for our annual All-Women's Camping Trip. We have all worked outside the home and we have talked about jobs, bosses, co-workers, and sexual harassment. Some of us had our babies together. We talked about breastfeeding, teething, and toilet training. We complained about our husbands. Later, we had issues with the school system or with rebellious teenagers. We cried and worried when our children left for college. We shared our cranky menopause years together and had a few campouts that weren't much fun. We helped each other through the deaths of our parents. Now our own aging is a big topic.

This group has spent many days and nights on the Platte River, a shallow, braided river that meanders across our state and is known for being "a mile wide and an inch deep." But it isn't always shallow. In the spring, bolstered with snowmelt from the Rockies, the Platte roars with ice jams crashing against each other in strong currents. In summer, when it rains a lot, the Platte can be a muddy swimming hole.

When I picture our river journey, I see my friends talking and laughing along the Platte. As with any other journey, every new day offers us surprises, danger, and tests of our courage, intelligence, and resolve. We encounter shoals and logjams as well as elderberry blossoms, lush sunsets, and the calls of wild geese.

Over the years my friends and I have discovered many empty, wild places. Invariably, when we get lost or something goes wrong, one of us reminds the others, "Remember the first rule of the wilderness: don't panic."

That is a good rule to keep in mind as we journey along our own rivers of time. If we can keep our wits about us, think clearly, and manage our emotions skillfully, we will experience a joyous time in our lives. If we have planned carefully and packed properly, if we have good maps and guides, the journey can be transcendent.

PART I

CHALLENGES
OF THE
JOURNEY

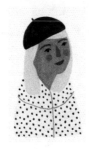

CHAPTER I

A New Stretch of the River

"The trouble is that old age is not interesting until one gets there, a foreign country with an unknown language to the young, and even to the middle-aged." —May Sarton

"The purpose of life, after all, is to live it, to taste experience to the utmost, to reach out eagerly and without fear for newer and richer experience." —Eleanor Roosevelt

THERE ARE MANY lifetimes in a lifetime. I was born in the Missouri Ozarks in 1947 to parents who were just returning home from serving in the Navy during World War II. That puts me on the leading cusp of the Baby Boomer generation. I grew up in Beaver City, Nebraska, where my mother worked as the town's doctor. I was the oldest child in a big family. We lived on the edge of town, and I spent my days reading or playing by Beaver Creek.

As a teenager, I was a socially inept, gawky girl. I went to the Methodist church, where I earnestly signed a pledge to never drink, swear, smoke, or have sex outside of marriage. On my red record player, I played Broadway musicals such as *Camelot*, *South Pacific*, and *Flower Drum Song*. Later, in high school, I listened to Dave Brubeck and Stan Getz and yearned for the day I could forever escape the Midwest.

After high school, I attended the University of California at Berkeley, during a time when it was a beacon for freedom and exploration of all kinds. My brother lived in San Francisco and we listened to the Grateful Dead and Janis Joplin in Golden Gate Park and at the Fillmore and the Avalon. I studied Tarot, astrology, and Sufism and I learned to make homemade granola and yogurt. By the time I graduated, I had broken all of my Methodist Youth Fellowship pledges.

Since then I have experienced other lifetimes, all in Nebraska—as a graduate student in psychology, as a mother of young children, and as the wife of Jim, a psychologist and musician. I have worked as a therapist, writer, and speaker. For the last seventeen years I've experienced the great privilege of being a grandmother with my five grandchildren living nearby.

There is continuity between all these lives. I have always loved to be around family and close friends, to be outdoors, to take long walks, to swim, and to look at the sky. Ever since I was young I have found comfort in reading, and I've always liked to take care of people and animals.

But I can also see great discontinuities. I can barely remember the girl who owned lacy babydoll pajamas, danced the Twist, and read her white leather Bible before turning out the lights and listening to KOMA. The young psychologist who scraped together $200 to buy a plaid suit to wear when she testified in court feels like a stranger. It seems as if these earlier experiences happened to someone else.

Many of us were children in the '50s, teenagers in the '60s, and college age during the height of the Vietnam War. Now we are in a new century and a new life stage, aware of how vulnerable everything is, including ourselves.

The only constant in the universe is change. The one thing we can predict about our own lives is that they will be unpredictable. In this life stage, we will be beset by internal and external crises.

When transitions happen and identities change, one of our great challenges is to find a new sense of meaning and purpose in our lives. That sounds simple but it isn't easy. As my doctor brother observed when he retired for health reasons, "You can't just go out and buy a pound of purpose." John is exactly right. We construct meaning when we choose what to do, how to help, and what stories to tell ourselves.

Of course, we need not be purposeful every day. Some days we may want to luxuriate in sleeping in, seeing friends, or watching movies. It's a question of balance and contrast. We do best when we learn how to have both work and rest in our lives.

In some ways, women are luckier than men because familiar roles hold our lives in place. We continue to do household chores, care for family, and see our friends. And many of us experience what Margaret Mead called "PMZ," post-menopausal zest. Yet to meet the challenges of this life stage, we must develop new habits. It is never too late to do this. In fact, we can't learn any younger.

As we age, our bodies and relationships change and the pace of change accelerates. At seventy we are unlikely to be able to function as we did in our fifties. We require fresh visions, better navigational skills, and new paradigms for framing our experiences. What worked yesterday will not be sufficient for tomorrow.

Change may be gradual, but our realization of it comes in bursts. Ava's watershed moment came when she was purchasing a ticket to the Art Institute of Chicago. The young man at the desk asked her if she wanted the senior citizen discount. That wasn't the usual response of men to Ava. She was a curvaceous brunette who always had been appealing to men. How could this man see her as a senior citizen?

On one level, of course, she knew she was sixty-five, but at the same time, she still saw herself as a gorgeous woman in her thirties. Her husband and many of the men she knew still treated her this way. It was strangers and newcomers who somehow couldn't see the thirty-year-old Ava. She didn't miss the catcalls as she walked down the street, but she did interpret men's silence to mean she was no longer attractive. That hurt.

The young man's remark knocked her back a step. She put her hand to her heart and waited for her breath to return. Then she said she wanted the discount.

Ava is an intelligent woman who knows that there is more to life than sexuality and beauty, but these have been critical pieces of her identity. As she sees her attractiveness fade, she feels disoriented. Ava told me, "I can't see myself as plain and forgettable. That's not who I am."

A developmental perspective in our sixties and seventies allows for a new openness in our hearts and minds. When we limit our belief in our own potential to grow, we also limit our incentive to grow. With the mind-set that abilities and talents can be developed, every place we go becomes our school and every person we meet becomes our teacher. The challenges and joys of this stage are catalytic. We can see the love in our friends' faces, taste the rain, and hear the song of the meadowlarks. We can do this even when we are walking out of a funeral or in pain from arthritis.

Resilience is not a fixed trait and we can master the skill of resilience in the same ways we learn to cook, drive, or do yoga. Growth isn't inevitable. Some women remain locked in their smallest selves cosseted by blankets of familiar but outdated ideas. Others wither emotionally over time and deal with life's many body blows by becoming more isolated and self-involved.

As Austrian novelist Marie von Ebner-Eschenbach wrote, "Old age transfigures or fossilizes." We all have encountered someone who complains constantly, talks only about herself, or is critical of others and unable to be self-aware. Sometimes we are these women. We all get grouchy, blue, and make uninspired choices. We lose battles with our appetites and impulses. However, it is never too late for us to do better.

We can grow in moral imagination. This increased capacity for empathy comes from our own suffering and our witness of suffering. Pain drives us deeper and makes us kinder. It also toughens us up. We can learn to withstand the roughest of currents. We can be profiles in courage. This is not a theoretical point. I've seen it happen to my clients, my friends, and my family members.

When I published *Reviving Ophelia*, my daughter was in high school and my therapy caseload was full of teenage girls in various degrees of pain, anger, and rebellion. I wanted to explore the cultural challenges to girls as they moved through this developmental stage. Now my daughter is forty and I have teenage granddaughters. As a gray-haired woman, I am confronting the cultural challenges of my own life stage.

Just as teenage girls can no longer rest in the womb of family, we older women can no longer be protected by the security of being young, healthy, and part of the ordinary flow of life. Both teenagers and older adults must craft for themselves a place in society with new responsibilities and goals. And they must cope with a radically changing body and a new set of expectations and cultural stereotypes.

When I told my adolescent granddaughter Kate about this book, I stressed that every life stage is hard. Looking back across my life decade by decade, I cannot find one that is without anguish.

Kate and I are both dealing with challenges now. I have health issues and attend frequent funerals of friends. Kate, just starting high school after being homeschooled, is encountering students and teachers with divergent points of view. She is developing a taste for new kinds of music and literature and learning more about the world and who she is. Kate is an enthusiastic and well-adjusted teenager, and I expect she will make good choices. But she won't have an easy time of it. No one her age does.

I told Kate that when I was younger I struggled with relationships more than I do now. I didn't know how to modulate my emotions or my passions. I worried about finding an intimate partner for life, choosing a career, and supporting a family. I said that I am also happier now than when my children were teenagers or during my most successful years as a writer when I was on the road and always feeling rushed, anxious, and exhausted.

At seventy, I am calmer and more settled, but only in retrospect does my life look organized and focused. Most of my life, I've been confused about what would happen next. Luck and chance have often been determinate. With information I had at the time, I made one choice after another. I couldn't have anticipated the outcome of many of those choices.

All life stages present us with joys and miseries. Fate and circumstance influence which stage is hardest for any given individual. But attitude and intentionality are the governors of the process. This journey can be redemptive if we find ways to grow from the struggles the stage offers us. Just as adolescents must find their North Stars to guide them, so must we elders maintain clarity about the kind of women we want to be.

Our development is fueled by the need to adapt to new circumstances. Time passes so quickly that our lives feel as fading as jet contrails. We are constantly engaged in a process of reflecting and problem solving. We ask questions such as "Now that I have time to travel, where do I want to go?" "Since my best friend moved to Arizona, whom do I call for a movie date?" "With my bad back, how do I carry in thirty-pound containers of birdseed?"

Simultaneously we explore the largest of questions. Did I make good use of my time and my talents? Am I now? Was I loving? Am I now? Was I loved? Am I now? What is my place in the universe?

As we seek answers we can make choices about our attitudes. For many of us, a combination of suffering and happiness is what defines this life stage and fuels our growth—we can describe ourselves as living in "both/and" terms. Suffering gives us empathy, while happiness gives us hope and energy. The contradictions of this life stage make it a portal for expanding our souls.

• • •

AT SEVENTY-TWO, WILLOW is fit and stylish with dark brown eyes and wavy auburn hair. She is at the peak of a long and satisfying career in human services. She is the only daughter of Russian immigrant parents who died when they were in their sixties, her father of a stroke and her mother of a heart attack.

Willow expected that she might die in her sixties. Ironically, her fear contributed to her excellent health. She never smoked or drank excessively or used drugs. She ate healthy foods and exercised over her lunch hours. She's always felt twenty years younger than her age. Her husband, Saul, still tells her she is pretty and she almost believes him.

Even before her parents' deaths, Willow had been deeply aware of life's finitude. Her parents often spoke of relatives who died as children or young adults. Many in her family were killed in pogroms and during World War II. Her father once told her that Jews were the people who truly understood the sanctity of time.

Yet, self-care only can go so far. Saul is slowing down and Willow knows she cannot continue to head the nonprofit where she works much longer. Her board of directors will want young leadership. It isn't good public relations to have an eighty-year-old director. Many of the contacts Willow cultivated have died or retired. Younger people are making the good contacts now. They have the energy for twelve-hour workdays.

However, Willow only knows how to work. Her sense of identity is almost identical to her sense of competence. Her parents worked long days in their cigar store and expected her to do the same at school. She studied from dawn to midnight and was class valedictorian in high school and at City College.

Ever since childhood in her poor neighborhood, Willow had dreamed of working with the homeless or other disadvantaged people. She studied social work in college and, right after she graduated, she found a job at a mental health center. Willow's boss both flirted with her and condescended to her, but she liked the clients. Soon she was running her own program and no longer had a boss who harassed her.

After college and two years of work, under some pressure from her family, Willow married her college sweetheart. He was fun and ambitious, but he wanted children and a traditional home life. When he started making money, he expected Willow to have a baby and stop working. Willow had no interest in that, and they divorced after two years.

Years later, Saul and Willow met at Saul's antiquarian bookstore. They shared a love of Russian literature and history. After a couple of years of conversations about books, Saul asked Willow out. They were in their fifties when they married. Saul was much more independent than her first husband and a cultured, gentle man. This time around, Willow made it clear that work came first.

Her current life is just what she wants. She and Saul live in a one-bedroom apartment near Central Park. It's close to her office and feels like a solarium. Willow had grown up in a small basement apartment under her parent's cigar store and luxury to her means light and space.

She loves dressing in a crisp business suit and going into her corner office in an old building on Ninety-Fourth Street. Usually she is at her desk by seven and she often stays until seven at night. She keeps her office door open and knows all the names of her clients with mental health issues. She brings every member of her staff pastries on their birthdays. Some of the clients, such as Ruby, the homeless baton twirler, and Myron, the man who thought he was vice president, feel like family members. She has cared for them for decades.

Once Saul had asked her if she could come home earlier. Willow snapped at him, "I'll come home when my work is done."

Saul waited a few months, then one evening while he rubbed Willow's shoulders he asked, "Wouldn't it be fun to travel and enjoy the cultural life of the city? If you aren't ready to retire, I wonder if you could cut down to half-time."

Willow felt a shiver of dread surge up her spine. She told him, "To me, retirement is the ugliest word in the English language."

Depending on her focus, Willow can describe herself as happy or sorrowful. She can emphasize her current prosperous life or her childhood poverty, her excellent health or her parents' early deaths, and her work satisfactions or her husband's desires that she cut back.

Willow no longer runs up six flights of stairs or remembers the names of everyone she meets. Most days she is positive and energetic, but sometimes, especially in the middle of the night, she panics about the future. She cannot stand the thought of being helpless or enfeebled.

• • •

LIKE WILLOW, NONE of us can stop time but, unless we have lost our capacity to think and cope, we have the potential to will ourselves into a good new place. With attitude and gratitude, we adapt. Furthermore, if we have been resilient people all of our lives, we are almost certain to respond to the inevitable changes of this era in skillful ways.

Even with the loss of beloved life partners, most women eventually recover. Soon after my co-worker Sarah's husband died, she told me, "I am walking around in a fugue state. I am acting in a play called *My New Life*. I will never be happy again."

Sarah suffered terribly the first two years alone. She needed medication to sleep and felt as fragile as a Fabergé egg. Her mantra during that time was "If you are walking through hell, keep walking." Five years later, Sarah is once again enjoying her life. She has even gone on a few dates. She said recently, "I've learned to never say never."

Those who do not suffer become insufferable. Our depth comes from experiencing a wide range of emotions, including profound tragedy, and our strength comes from that which could destroy us. As we grow from heartbreak, we increase our pain tolerance. As my friend Nora put it, "Leona's death prepared me for my son's burn accident, and that prepared me for this terrible moment when my sister is dying. I know how hard life can be, so I enjoy every good day."

Without suffering, too much is taken for granted. With a transcendent response to suffering, nothing is too small to appreciate. We can enjoy every fresh apricot, blazing October day, and visit with a friend. We can be awake and whole.

Of course, all of this is easier said than done. None of us manages a transcendent response with everything. This book is not promoting perfection, but rather engagement in a process that will make us happier.

My premise is that there is an amazing calculus at play in this developmental stage. The more that is taken from us, the more capacity we have for compassion and appreciation. Growth requires healing from tragedies and integrating them into our own wholeness. Though we have lost a great deal, we can strive to become women who experience a great appreciation for life.

One of the great paradoxes of this life stage is that we experience not only the largest number of catastrophes but also the highest well-being. Our contentment comes from acceptance of life as it is. Wisdom compensates for our travails. We can navigate the river's snags, logjams, and downpours with competence and confidence. We can explore the mysteries along the river of time that we help each other travel down.

I was most aware both of the powers of others to help me and my own power to find what I needed in the winter of 2017. During the week of Donald Trump's inauguration as president, I attended a retreat at Ghost Ranch in New Mexico with noted Buddhist teacher Joanna Macy. She had gathered earth protectors together to help us prepare for the future. We spoke of our fears, sorrows, and anger in the face of terrible news about Mother Earth and climate change. We cried together and we also danced and sang together.

One clear morning we were encouraged to walk outside and look for something that spoke to us. Then we could sit down with that particular object and observe it carefully. After this, we were to design a small ceremony involving the object.

As I walked over the semi-frozen red dirt, I wore a heavy winter coat, gloves, and hiking boots. I could see the great Chama Valley, where the Tewa people had lived for centuries. A silver river wound through this valley and right up to Ghost Ranch. Rising above the valley were the bloodred, orange, and pink Sangre de Cristo Mountains that looked exactly as Georgia O'Keeffe had painted them.

Two ravens were squawking on a dead branch, and a flurry of wrens, like Christmas decorations, adorned a piñon pine. Chamisa rabbitbrush sparkled in the sunlight. Almost everything spoke to me. But I walked on for a while, listening to my footsteps on the crunchy ground, breathing the pure mountain air, and wondering what my significant object would be.

As I approached Ghost Ranch's labyrinth, I spotted it. Without any conscious thought, I knew this was it. The change in my breathing told me. On the high bank above the gurgling arroyo stood a large cholla cactus covered with bright yellow pears and thorns. Her pale green arms stretched Shiva-like in all directions. She was old and tattered with some of her branches blackened and withered. At the same time, a few new appendages of a rich purple color were sprouting. That was exactly how I felt about myself. The starry-eyed high school girl, the young mother of a newborn, and even the woman who could ice-skate and cross-country ski had perished. Yet I also could feel new rich growth rising within me.

I sat on the cold ground by this battered cactus for some time. Behind it white clouds skittered by and disappeared. New clouds formed. After a while, the elements of my ceremony revealed themselves.

I pricked my finger with a thorn and offered my blood to all my ancestors and the ancestors of other living beings who had created this magnificence. I leaned over and gingerly kissed the top of a yellow pear.

I realized that this cactus with its withered arms symbolized what my life would be. It would consist of thorns and fruit, pain and beauty. My body would age; my soul would expand.

CHAPTER 2

The Lay
of the Land

"*I deserve better*—such a dangerous, mad thought for a
woman to entertain." —Meredith Duran

"Women may be the one group that grows more
radical with age." —Gloria Steinem

ONE FALL AFTERNOON I sat in Holmes Park with a bird guide and bino-
culars. A little girl with blond curls and a red wool cap approached me
for a look at my book. As her mother watched, I showed the little girl
some pictures of ducks and geese and pointed out their resemblance to
the birds we could see on the lake. The little girl enjoyed this, but after
I closed the bird book she looked at me and asked with sincerity and
kindness, "Where do old ladies come from?" Apparently, she thought we
were a separate species!

Older people are walking reminders that aging is everyone's inevitable fate. In our society, we see cultural and emotional distancing from

the old. Of course, this causes distress to both sexes, but women can be especially disempowered.

Old women in America suffer a social disease. For us, ageism may be an even more serious challenge than aging. Our sexuality is mocked, our bodies are derided, and our voices are silenced. We can feel as useless as poinsettias a week after Christmas. In a society that values the young, fit, and beautiful, we all eventually wind up lacking. To make it even worse, older women, including witches and mothers-in-law, are often portrayed as evil villains, intent on doing harm. Although some women have reappropriated the word "crone" and utilized it for empowerment, the population at large does not value crones.

Birthday cards for older women are demeaning. Their jokes are about being senile, drinking too much, or being either sexually over-the-hill or sexually insatiable. While jokes about different races are considered impolite and harmful, jokes about old women are not taboo. In fact, they are everywhere.

When I tell my friends that I'm writing a book about older women, they often respond indignantly. "I'm not old." "Old" is a negative word in our culture, like "fat" or "dirty." What women mean when they say, "I am not old," is "I won't accept the ideas that the culture has about me."

Television, movies, fashion, and advertising rarely reflect the needs and circumstances of older women. A February 2017 joint study by the Media Diversity and Social Change Initiative and Humana found that older people appeared in fewer than 12 percent of all Academy Award–winning movies between 2014 and 2016. Furthermore, almost none of these older people were women. The Geena Davis Institute on Gender in Media reports that in family films, male characters outnumber female characters by three to one. With some notable exceptions, women over forty have gone missing in Hollywood.

Everywhere in America, attractiveness is overvalued as a defining characteristic. Women's bodies, no matter how old, are expected to look young and slender. The older we get, the harder it is to meet this ideal. Meanwhile, in this culture, many of our strengths, such as caretaking, emotional processing, peacemaking, and connecting to others, are not acknowledged.

I recently met a beautiful woman my age who works in publishing. Rosa told me she did not want to dye her hair brown, but she had been warned she needed to look young in order to keep her job. Many older women experience great pressure to look young and often consider cosmetic surgery. But we are damned if we do and damned if we don't.

If we forego cosmetic surgery, we may risk losing our jobs or our partners. Yet, if we undergo cosmetic surgery and it doesn't go well, we feel even less attractive and also deeply humiliated. We may be mocked. Even when it does go well, most women keep cosmetic surgery a secret. They don't want to be judged for artificially improving their looks, or trying to appear younger.

Older women are sometimes perceived as incompetent. My seventy-five-year-old cousin, who still holds a full-time job, was paying for her groceries at the checkout line when the cashier inflicted help by offering advice on what money she should pull out of her wallet. My cousin said that she was torn between laughing at the absurdity of the situation, bursting into tears, or telling her that she could still manage cash just fine.

Another unpleasant experience is when people address us with the plural pronoun, such as "Do we want our jacket now, honey?" or "What do we want for our breakfast?" Ha ha. That use of "we" is infantilizing and can send some of us around the bend.

Explanations for the behavior of the old tend to be markedly different from what they are for the behavior of younger people. For example, if an older woman has a fender bender or gets a speeding ticket, it may be attributed to the fact that she is old. Some of us are not good drivers, no question about that. On the other hand, it could have been the kind of accident anyone could have. If a younger woman had experienced it, the assumption would be that she was in a hurry or just unlucky, or it might be shrugged off by saying, "Everyone makes mistakes."

These unfair judgments can come up around finances. If we have an overdraft or an unbalanced checkbook, we may be vulnerable to a discussion of our money-managing capabilities. Getting lost, leaving the stove on, and falling have different implications when we are old.

Not long ago a friend in his twenties came over to plant butterfly milkweed with me. We had a good talk while we worked, and I felt satisfied with our visit. That is, until I went in and looked in the mirror. I could see salsa on my shirt. Immediately I was chagrined and wondered if my young friend would think that I was getting addled. If I had been younger, I would not have entertained that thought.

As we age, we also experience role reversals that can feel disempowering. Younger people have the prestige and prominence. Our supervisors, doctors, and attorneys are sometimes decades younger than we are. Our adult children are moving into their own power and, in many cases, they do not want our advice and opinions. This is no one's fault, but it changes power relationships in ways that can be confusing and painful.

If we're not careful, we can internalize negative messages and feel ashamed of our bodies, our wrinkles, and our assigned roles. We may struggle with valuing ourselves and even make derogatory comments about ourselves and other older women. Negative cultural scripts can become self-fulfilling prophecies. If we are told we are worthless, we can become worthless. If we are told we are not capable of a rich and enjoyable life, we may not build that life for ourselves.

Young people do not understand older people because they have never been old. When we are old, we have memories of being a child, a teenager, a young adult, or a middle-aged person. Our own experiences provide us with a vehicle for empathy and understanding. Younger people have no frame of reference for the experience of sixty-year-olds. They cannot quite imagine our felt reality.

In 2012, the Yale School of Public Health conducted a study of social disapproval of the old in Facebook groups. They found that in the twenty-to-twenty-nine-year-old age group, 75 percent of participants denigrated older people. This study talked at length about what they called "gerontophobia" and its implications for social policy. Of course, ultimately ageism is a prejudice against one's own future self.

Margaret Mead defined an ideal society as one with a place for every human gift. Our cultural scripts do not offer aging women much of a place. The stories of our complexity, our wisdom, and our joy are not often told.

This isn't true in every culture. When immigrants and refugees arrive in our country, some find work in nursing homes and assisted living facilities. They are often surprised by how older people are treated here. These newcomers often come from places where old people are cared for by their families and tribes.

Around the world, when countries industrialize, the relationships between parents and children change rapidly. In Thailand, young people from the villages have moved into the cities for work and left old people behind. For the first time in Thai history, older people have no one to help them. In Japan, there is a long tradition of living with and caring for aging parents, but this is changing as adults of both sexes work long hours and live in small apartments in crowded cities. Japanese young adults have neither room for their parents to live with them nor time to care for them. This has now become a crisis in Japan.

In our culture, we don't have useful language to talk about the relationship between generations. Our ideas about independence and dependency lead us to see the world in an either/or way. Older women fear being dependent and children want to be independent. Neither one of these concepts reflects reality. In fact, we are all interdependent all of the time.

If we could think of ourselves as interdependent, as people who are both cared for and care for others, then we could reconceptualize the interactions between the old and the young. Younger people would be more appreciative of what we have to offer. Older people could see themselves as part of a circle of caring that begins with our oldest living relatives and flows down to the youngest baby.

Many older people have almost no contact with the young and vice versa. This is unfortunate for individuals, families, and the culture as a whole. When generations interact, cultures tend to flourish. The different age groups inspire and energize each other. When we understand our interconnectedness, we value each other's gifts. Otherwise, we base our opinions on the stereotyped stories that abound in our culture. A great deal of potential is lost.

There are notable exceptions to age-related segregation. Many of us have young friends. Some people are not ageist. We often experience younger people stepping up with offers to help. On a recent trip to Chicago, young men and women offered to put my carry-on luggage overhead in the plane and, later, to take it down for me. On the crowded train into the city, a teenager immediately offered me his seat. Walking up a long flight of stairs into my hotel lobby, I was stopped by a young woman who offered to carry my suitcase up the stairs. This kindness and respect for the old always brings me to tears. I am so grateful. So honored.

Many older women report that, as they shop, work, volunteer, or exercise, they are simply not noticed by younger people. An attorney friend told me that, when she is in line for customer service or to order food, younger people often walk in front of her up to the counter. If she is with her husband buying appliances, furniture, or a car, sales clerks address him. She said, "I'm invisible now. I could take off all my clothes and walk through the courthouse and I'm not sure anyone would notice."

Parenthetically, invisibility is not always unpleasant. It can sometimes be freeing. When we are not noticed, we can behave however we want. We can be good observers of what is going on around us. With invisibility, we have permission not to worry so much about appearances or proper behavior. We can be silly, quirky, and free to do as we please. If we aren't working, we don't need to dress for success. As Emma from Denver put it, "I don't have one pair of pants that I bought in this millennium."

If we want to, we can live in sweatpants and T-shirts. We can skip events that we don't care to attend. But while invisibility may sometimes work in our favor, ageism never does, especially when we possess it ourselves.

I interviewed Suzanna in the cafeteria at the hospital where she worked. She was a tall, angular woman dressed in a mustard-colored suit with matching shoes. We had lived in the same community for years, but this was our first meeting. I had heard her described as "the most confident woman I know" and "a natural leader." Suzanna had a friendly smile, but a brisk manner that signaled, "Let's get to work."

We jumped right into a discussion of stereotyping. Suzanna said that she worked on an administrative team where she was the oldest woman in her group. She found herself hiding her age and signaling that she was as young as her co-workers. She said, "I want to own my age. However, if I reveal how old I am, it comes with so much baggage."

She confessed that, even though she was sixty-nine, she held the same negative image of older women that young people did. When she read in the obituaries that someone had died at age sixty-nine or seventy, she would think, "Well, at least they were old." But then, she would realize, "No. Wait. Holy crap, that's my age. I am not ready to die."

Suzanna noted that in the past few months she had felt less confident when she gave presentations in large meetings. She wondered if she had as strong a voice or as energetic a performance as she once had. She looked at me quizzically. "Am I crazy to feel that way?" We both laughed, but not gleefully.

She lifted her coffee mug with both hands and took a slow sip. Then she told me her job was meaningful and she liked working; however, the hospital required mandatory retirement at age seventy. Suzanna was accustomed to being recognized for her work and she wondered how she would feel when that recognition was gone. She said, "My retired friends do not receive much praise. I guess their validation must come from within."

Suzanna had become a strong feminist in college. Even though she was in a decades-long relationship with an artist named Walt, her identity was never centered on attractiveness or her relationship with a man. She belonged to a community of close women friends and delighted in all kinds of activities. She felt curious about her many new emotions and identity issues, such as the fact that she was now the oldest woman in her neighborhood. She laughed, "Somehow, I always felt that growing old happened to other people."

When her mother was alive, Suzanna befriended many of the residents at the assisted living facility where her mom lived. Now twice a month she drives there to lead a bingo game. This experience has challenged her stereotypes of older people. She described one older woman who occasionally nods off during bingo. Suzanna had considered her senile, but now understands that, when this woman is awake, she converses with animation and humor.

As we finished our coffees, we returned to the great disconnect between stereotypes and what she thinks and feels. She said, "Walt and I just saw a movie with great singing and dancing, but, with a cast of hundreds, there was not one older woman actor. It was as if the ideal world would not have us in it."

I agreed, "No wrinkles or arm flab in that movie." We shared another mirthless laugh as she waved goodbye.

Suzanna is doing her best to cope with cultural ideas about older women. Even with her feminist background, leadership role, and community work, she has discovered that fighting ageism, even in herself, is a tough slog.

In *Reviving Ophelia* I wrote about America's stories for teenage girls. The reality of their lives is so much more complicated and interesting than the cultural scr   that define them. Unlike adolescents, who are just entering t┌   ┐der society, we older women have lived in it for decades. Our   s are fully mature and most of us have developed skills in analyzing, advocating, and educating. But even with our maturity, we must see our constraints in order to break free from them.

Meridel Le Sueur wrote, "Survival is resistance." Because our current cultural stories about how we should behave are useless, we have great freedom to throw off our chains and resist definition by the broader culture.

My favorite story of resistance comes from a book called *Two Old Women* by Velma Wallis. In it she retells the legend of the Athabaskan tribe in Alaska. One cold winter when their community was starving, two ancient women were left behind. The male elders felt they could not feed people who were unable to work. The women had nothing but their clothing, a leather bag for boiling food, and a hatchet that one of the women's grandsons secretly had left for her. The women expected they would die soon. The old ones always did. But the younger woman argued, "Why don't we try to stay alive? Maybe we can make it. I'd rather die trying."

The older woman agreed and the two women become self-sufficient. They struggled with hunger, freezing temperatures, and lack of shelter, but managed to walk to a slough that they remembered as children. They camped along this slough, fished, and hunted for rabbits and squirrels. Not only did they survive, but eventually they were able to catch and dry many fish. After several weeks, their starving tribe happened upon their hut and the old women were able to share their stash of supplies. After that, the women were much revered by the Athabaskans and their story was told for generations. It's a beautiful true story about what determined women can do.

We can claim our power and secure respect for older women in three primary ways. First, we can take responsibility for educating other people about both the negative stereotypes and the reality of our lives. We can resolve not to criticize ourselves or other women or make negative remarks about aging or appearance. We can state out loud, "I don't like mother-in-law jokes" or "What you just said about older women doesn't mesh with the women I know."

We can be advocates for women of all ages, working to create the institutions and policies we require to live healthy, social, and productive lives throughout the life span. We can dismantle ageist policies and practices with lobbying, letter-writing campaigns, legal action, and protests. There is nothing that grabs the attention of the press more quickly than older women demonstrating with props such as rocking chairs or bouquets of wildflowers. We can write, speak out, or utilize music, art, and theater to change the way we are treated and perceived.

Finally, we can converse with people of all ages. We can visit with whomever we meet as we run errands or take a walk. We can compliment parents when we see them doing a good job. We can praise young workers in restaurants or grocery stores on their work ethic. If they are doing a good job, we can ask, "Who taught you how to work this way?"

Younger and older women working together is a great way to facilitate mutual respect, empathy, and understanding. We can unite with younger women around particular causes or projects. We can form educational groups together and study what we need to learn to be more effective advocates. We can go together to legislators and other policymakers to lobby for causes of importance to all of us.

Especially when we act together, we can create power out of thin air. Advocacy for a broader understanding of women in our life stage will not only benefit us, but it will benefit all generations to come.

The culture shapes us and we shape it. In a society that values young female beauty, older women lose status as they gain years. As our bodies grow old, we must find new ways to stay engaged and empowered. We must both care for our aging bodies and teach the culture to care about us. Let's push into the current and row.

CHAPTER 3

The Worn Body

"Dread of one's own aging leads to fear and dislike of old people, and the fear feeds upon itself. In Western society, this cycle of dread has been going on a long, long time."
—Alexandra Robbin

"We wither, sag, wrinkle, crinkle, tatter, and become marked by life's events. Time and gravity, air and water wear us down, each into a unique and precious beauty, every bit as beautiful as a landscape or plant weathered by the seasons."
—Stephanie Sugars

SOMETIMES MY FRIEND Pia feels a compulsion to take visitors into her study and say, "I was young once." She shows them a photograph of herself at the University of Chicago in 1969. She's in a garden, surrounded by leafy green trees, wearing a psychedelic shirt and a paisley headband over her long blond curls. Her cheeks are rounded and smooth; her eyes are flashing and her lips are full and rosy. Pia wants others to know that she was not always the gray-haired, wrinkled, and thin woman she is now.

As we move toward our seventies, our bones, shape, vision, sense of smell and taste, and even our teeth change. We react differently to medications. We don't tolerate the cold as well. As our skin thins, we bruise more easily and our cartilage deteriorates. We struggle with our balance and coordination. Everything seems to droop and sag.

Women who have previously felt attractive and sexy often experience a crisis of confidence. They look in the mirror and now see wrinkles. Even if they are thin, they have flab. One of my friends stopped wearing a swimsuit at age forty. She said, "I don't want to ruin anyone's day at the beach." Another considered cosmetic surgery for her sagging neck, but then decided that she'd rather spend the money on a trip to Hawaii. Good for her.

Our sexuality changes in surprising ways. Some women experience diminished interest in sexual activity, while others become more sexual. Rita, who has always been a highly sexual person, no longer has much desire for sex. On the other hand, Millie's trust for her partner of forty years helps her relax and enjoy sex more than ever. Illness, isolation, and loneliness also have their effects on sexual appetites and experiences.

• • •

Sylvia and Lewis live in a small home in Austin, Texas, with their two custodial grandchildren. Before their retirement, Sylvia worked as a paralegal and Lewis was an electrician. He still takes odd jobs now and then to supplement their income. They belong to a small Evangelical church near their home.

When Sylvia smiles, there is a gap between her two front teeth; but Sylvia doesn't smile as often as she used to. She was born with a sunny disposition, but the last twenty years have taken a toll. The jokester in her has gone to sleep. Sylvia has a limp from childhood polio and painful arthritis. She is heavy and doesn't have the time or energy for an exercise routine. She can't afford a gym membership.

Sylvia and Lewis have one daughter, Lenore. They raised her in their church and paid for piano lessons for her. Until high school, Lenore was doing all right except for her grades, but then she started drinking, using drugs, and staying out all night. Before graduation she dropped out of school and lived on the streets. Lenore was first addicted to methamphetamines and then moved on to heroin. Sylvia and Lewis have spent a great deal of their savings on unsuccessful drug treatment and rehabilitation programs for Lenore.

Having a daughter who is mentally ill has been the worst experience of Sylvia's life. She told me, "You don't know what scared is until you have a daughter who is drug addicted, homeless, and incommunicado."

Lenore is still using and Sylvia doesn't know where she is. The last time she heard from Lenore, she was in Oklahoma City in a halfway house. When Sylvia tried to call there, the number had been disconnected.

After they lost Lenore, Lewis became much more introverted. Sylvia encouraged him to go fishing or play cards on Friday nights with his friends. But instead he watched television every night and often fell asleep in his recliner. Sylvia and her Lewis once had a lively sexual relationship. However, they haven't had sex in years. Sylvia crawled into bed by herself and many mornings woke up alone.

Sylvia couldn't help Lewis through the grief process. She could barely make coffee in the morning and drive herself to work. She stopped seeing her friends because she felt she detected pity on their faces. No one knew what to say to her. After she finished with dinner and the dishes at night, she would go to her bedroom and look at pictures of Lenore and cry. She suspected Lewis was crying, too, but unfortunately, they cried in separate rooms.

Now in their late sixties, they are caring for Lenore's children. Max is ten and has some learning disabilities. He is a tall, skinny kid with big ears and the same gap between his teeth that his grandmother has. Gracie is eight and a good-natured girl. She is plump and wears her hair in tight braids that stick out on top of her head. Both children are full of energy and requests. Sylvia told Lewis, "God caused menopause for a reason. He knew sixty-year-olds were too old to raise children."

Sylvia rarely talked about her arthritis pain and she didn't take medication. Her long-term physician recently retired and Sylvia missed him. He had attended her church, and they often exchanged vegetables and homemade relishes.

Eventually Sylvia's pain inspired her to make an appointment with a new doctor. At her first appointment, she felt uneasy. Dr. Peterson was younger and he looked at his computer more than he looked at her.

He chided her on her weight and lack of exercise. He told her that her blood pressure and cholesterol were too high and he recommended lifestyle changes, especially more exercise. At the end of the appointment he informed Sylvia he didn't prescribe opioids because they were too addictive. Instead, he wrote an order for a pain clinic.

When she left Sylvia felt angry and discouraged. She had no intention of going to a pain clinic. She was too busy caring for the grandchildren and they didn't have the money for therapy. If they had more extra income, they would spend it on dental implants for Lewis.

Sylvia grumbled to herself about how unlikely it was that, at her age and under stress, she would be able to make significant "lifestyle changes." She thought, "If the doctor's life were like mine, when would he exercise? Would he want to give up enchiladas for dinner or the comfort of a chocolate bar at the end of the day?"

• • •

As we age, even those of us with better situations than Sylvia's sense that our energy is flagging. We may still want to do big garden projects or walk the length of Manhattan, but our bodies beg us not to. We wake with a strong life force, but after a few hours, it fades. A common question is, "How did we manage to do everything we used to do?"

We all must bid goodbye to some of our physical pleasures. My friend Carmen no longer plays tennis. Leanne, a landscaper, no longer can meet the heavy demands her job requires. Abbie no longer can read and has switched to audiobooks.

Even our minds work differently. Our brains are more prone to falling into ruts. To our dismay, we discover that we no longer easily do five things at once. We can't quickly learn new languages or complex games such as chess. Many of us lose some short-term memory.

Most discussions about memory in older people concern deterioration and loss, but such discussions miss an important phenomenon. Our minds become less cluttered and more concerned with essentials. We develop deeper and more integrated memories. Where we put our cell phone or sunglasses is background. Foreground is a mix of memories about family, friends, history, turning points, and crucible moments.

We may forget details but we excel at retrieving stories. We have a lifetime of material to draw from. These memories can be useful for practical reasons: "My mother-in-law made the best piecrusts ever because she only used lard"; as a warning: "I remember what happened when my aunt appointed her boyfriend power of attorney"; for comfort: "When I have trouble sleeping, I remember what it felt like to sleep beside my children when they were babies"; as inspiration: "My parents made it through the Great Depression and World War II; surely I can make it through hard times as well"; and for moral clarity: "My mother said that good manners consisted of following the Golden Rule."

Like an old river, our memories run deep and clear. We can see the relationships between things that happened fifty years ago and the ways we react today. Our ability to make connections and distinctions grows stronger. We live more comfortably with complexity and multiple points of view.

We know, even when we are staggering from life's blows, that pain is a constant part of the human condition and that we are equipped to survive it. We learn to accept what will become a constant cycle of maintenance, loss, accommodation, and renewal.

When we were younger most of us took our health for granted. In graduate school I smoked Kool Menthols, drank coffee by the barrel, and ate sugary donuts for breakfast. Every weekend I drank wine with my friends, and my primary exercise was walking from the parking lot to the psychology building at the University of Nebraska. In the summer, I studied outside so I could soak in the sun. Still, I went years without needing a doctor. I didn't even have health insurance. Everything just worked.

I never thought that one day I would have cataract surgeries, osteoporosis, and multiple basal cell cancers. I didn't imagine my teeth would turn yellow. Now I wish I'd used more sunscreen and worked harder on my posture. I wish I hadn't smoked for twenty years.

As we age, we look at old people with kinder eyes. We gain a deeper understanding of our parents and grandparents. My father had a stroke when he was forty-nine. I was eighteen at the time and it didn't seem strange that my father would suffer a series of strokes and die at fifty-four. Of course, it was terribly sad but, after all, I considered him old. Now my son is forty-six, and I am twenty-one years older than my father was when he had his first stroke.

I remember chiding my mother for "walking like an old lady." She had suffered several tumbles on the ice and eventually purchased a four-pronged cane. Sometimes now, when I am walking on ice, I wish I had that cane.

When I was younger, I was bored and/or disgusted by any talk about health. Why on earth did my older relatives discuss gallbladders, problems with their bowels, and cataract surgeries? I could somewhat understand why these topics were important to the people suffering from them, but my relatives were also interested in the ailments of strangers.

I was shocked by how graphic and blunt older people were about their bodies. I remember once listening to an uncle tell us all about his swollen testicle. Another aunt talked about her constipation. Various adults elaborated on their trouble with sleeping. As a young girl, I could think of nothing duller than discussing sleep.

By now I have a different perspective. I also talk about health. I am still surprised when male friends tell me about the effects of chemo on their sex life or their issues with bladder control, but I am much less surprised now than I would have been even five years ago. Of course we talk about health. It is the major concern in many of our lives. If it were flooding outside, we'd talk about water.

Yet, these conversations are not always as dismal as they sound. We can learn to accommodate and even laugh at our troubles. Health talk can be couched in jokes and anecdotes about funny situations. Phyllis Diller was a master at this. "I'm at an age where my back goes out more than I do." One friend who is undergoing chemotherapy refers to herself as a "chemo sapien." My neighbor wins the award for the best sense of humor about adversity. She has had a double mastectomy and, on Halloween, she wears small matching pumpkins in her bra.

Yolanda's mother, Eve, was even able to make a joke just before she died. Eve had never been willing to use medication. She didn't trust over-the-counter drugs and, except for childbirth, she never visited a doctor. She lived a healthy lifestyle, did hard physical labor, and assumed she would die when the time came.

She was right about that. At ninety-eight, she contracted pneumonia, a disease my mother always called "the old person's friend." Eve was admitted to an ICU. She was in quite a lot of pain and a doctor offered her some morphine.

Eve started to shake her head no, then hesitated and nodded yes. The doctor gave her a shot and within seconds her body was relaxed. With a teasing smile, Eve said to Yolanda, "I've made a terrible mistake with my life. I should have taken drugs long ago."

They both laughed.

There is always the possibility of self-rescue. We can choose where to focus our attention and will our way to gratitude. At least we have needed medical care available! Whatever our situation, it could always be worse. It helps to envision that worst-case scenario and feel lucky to have escaped it.

Recently I went to a sidewalk café with Abby, who had just finished radiation and chemotherapy for her ovarian cancer. She told me that she no longer recognized herself. She felt like a shell, hollowed out inside with no markers left of the person she had been. She felt her personality had been drained from her by all of the treatments. But, just at that moment, a beautiful pot of herbal tea arrived with almond croissants. As she sipped the tea and nibbled on a croissant, she smiled and said, "The Abby who likes croissants is coming back to me."

• • •

KESTREL IS A short woman with frosty blue eyes and an equally frosty personality. She works in a technology company in Seattle. She lives alone in an apartment with a view of the Puget Sound.

Kestrel grew up in rural Washington in a conservative working-class family. Her father was an alcoholic and abusive. One night when her father was choking her mother, Kestrel hit him on the head with an iron and said she would kill him if he ever touched any of them again. Her father swore at her and then skulked away, but he never again hit anyone in the family.

Kestrel felt oddly grateful to her father. His cruelty gave her something hard to push against and allowed her to grow up emotionally sturdy. The strength she built opposing him, her desire to protect the vulnerable, and her scrappiness and grit had served her well. She was a member of Pride and was passionate about fighting injustice.

Unfortunately, other things had lasted too. She trusted no one but herself and formed only casual relationships. She was currently dating a teacher named Becca, but she maintained her emotional distance. She wouldn't let Becca stay the night and she never said "I love you." As with her father, Kestrel's primary relationship was with alcohol.

She had a crucible moment when she heard news about her health. When she had a bone scan at sixty-four, her doctor told her that she had osteoporosis. The doctor asked how much Kestrel drank; she told her that she usually drank a bottle of red wine a night. The doctor pursed her lips with worry and said that Kestrel needed to cut out alcohol and to start drinking milk. Kestrel groaned and said, "The last time I drank milk, I was in diapers."

They both laughed at that.

Kestrel asked what would happen if she didn't follow orders; her doctor said, "You'll end up fracturing your spine unloading a dishwasher or breaking a hip."

Kestrel gulped and looked away to steady herself. This news made her want a drink.

The doctor also advised her to stop any activities that involved risks of falling, including her favorite activity, cycling in the Cascades and the Olympic Mountains. Instead she suggested Kestrel lift weights.

When she left the doctor's office Kestrel was so angry she could spit. In addition to all the damage her father had inflicted on the family, he had bequeathed her his alcoholism. She swore as she walked down the street, and she stopped twice to kick tires. She kicked one tire so hard she hurt her foot. She limped home and called Becca to swear some more.

Kestrel did not even consider Alcoholics Anonymous. She hated the idea of being vulnerable around other people or sharing her thoughts and feelings about herself. However, Kestrel stopped drinking on her birthday. Fortunately, she had an iron will and could control everything except her temper.

For the first few months, she found it difficult to be with the Pride women who were drinking. It was also hard to abstain when she was home alone or at a sushi bar with co-workers. Nothing soothed her like alcohol did. However, her reflections on broken bones and spinal fractures motivated her to abstain. She had a lifetime of being strong and enduring frustration. Eventually, Kestrel found a substitute drink for dinners out: tonic water with lime. She managed to abstain, but she was tense and developed insomnia. She hadn't yet healed from the issues that made alcohol so seductive.

• • •

Working on my book about refugees, I learned a great deal about trauma and recovery, and with the help of the people I spoke with developed what I called "a healing package of treatments." These treatments could be medical interventions from Western doctors, traditional medicines from the refugee's culture of origin, or basic pleasures. For example, a common healing package for a refugee family included going to city parks, cooking foods from their homelands, and meeting people who spoke their language.

All of us can create our own healing packages by thinking about that which makes us feel healthy, calm, and happy. We can write our own prescriptions for health that include nutrition and exercise, relationships, things we enjoy, and gratitude.

I had my own opportunity to develop resilience in November of 2014, a bleak month for me. I learned that my brother's prostate cancer had returned after a six-year hiatus. My friend Marianne died and then, two weeks later, my friend Kent died. My dentist told me I needed a gum graft. Oh, and I found out my hands were badly damaged and almost worn out.

My hands had been stiff and sore and I scheduled an appointment with a physical therapist. I expected he would encourage me to ice them and take regular breaks. Instead, after an hour and a half of testing, he expressed surprise that I could cook, drive a car, or dress myself. Dan said, "Your hands need to be in a hospital."

He suggested I try hand-strengthening exercises and return in two weeks. He told me not to pick up my nine-month-old grandson, garden, or lift weights. He also said I could not type or handwrite another book. I asked Dan if I might outlive my hands if I overworked them. He responded, "That is how you need to think."

I shouldn't have been surprised. All of my life, I had been rough on my hands. At age ten I was working in my mother's office with heavy equipment as I sterilized syringes, non-disposable rubber gloves, and surgical equipment. By the time I was in high school, I was working full-time in the summer as a carhop at the A&W on Highway 81. I carried full trays of malts and hamburgers down the central runway. The last two years of high school I was a fry cook at that same A&W. That job required constant chopping and working with heavy fryers. In college and while working on my doctorate, I had written many hours a day. As a therapist, I had taken notes as I sat with clients. The last thirty years, I've worked on manuscripts for six to eight hours a day.

I shouldn't have been surprised, but I was shocked. I had always seen myself as a strong, healthy, and competent person. I held the belief that if I worked hard enough, I could pretty much do anything. I couldn't conceive of who I would be if I were not physically useful.

When I arrived home, I told my husband the news. He sat quietly for a while, then he said, "We'll make it through this."

Of course, I carried on. I had no choice. And I was lucky I could afford quality health care. I purchased the appropriate hand braces and canceled my yoga class. I exercised and hoped for some improvement.

I thought that if the gods had wanted to punish me, they couldn't have done a better job than to make me helpless. Yet, if the gods had wished to give me the largest possible point of view on the universe, this is exactly what my trial would be. When I told my gentle cousin Roberta that I thought the gods were testing me, she said firmly, "Leave the gods out of it. These things just happen to people."

There is a Chinese saying that all great knowledge comes from great pain, but the converse is not necessarily true. Not all pain leads to great knowledge. As a therapist, I had encouraged others to learn from their despair and pain. I was determined to do the same thing for myself. I knew I needed to end my argument with reality and grow into a person who could handle my new situation with gratitude.

After two weeks, I returned to Dan to be retested. My hand strength had not improved. Exercises would not help me. Heavy snow began to fall as I drove home. The icy road and whiteout seemed a painfully perfect metaphor for my inner landscape. Indeed, it felt as if the sky were crying snow.

That Saturday, Jim went to a friend's home to watch a football game. I stayed home alone at dusk and watched snow falling. Snow has always been evocative to me—even, I would say, spiritual. I needed to write about my despair. I knew that for the sake of my hands, I shouldn't write, but I told myself this was a "quality of life" exception. After a while, I had so many notes I decided to open a file folder on the topic of my hands.

I found a picture postcard of myself from promotional events for *Writing to Change the World*. I taped it on the cover of the folder and examined it. Suddenly, I was seized with rage and I grabbed a magic marker and slashed a big X across my face. The cover now basically said, *Mary Pipher: Not Writing to Change the World.*

I was surprised by my rage. For a while I just sat with my emotions. Hot waves of anger and pain swelled in my chest. Then all of a sudden, I burst out laughing at the irony of my situation.

With that, I was once again a writer. I recalled Bertolt Brecht's answer to the question, "In the dark times will there also be singing?" He responded, "Yes. There will also be singing about the dark times." That turning toward singing, or in my case writing, made all the difference.

Meanwhile, I learned how to use special tools in the kitchen and to hold a pen designed for damaged hands. My husband opened cans and jars and helped me pull up my socks. My son-in-law set up a dictation system for me. I played with the baby on the floor or when someone handed him to me.

Adjusting to this new normal was neither easy nor simple. Jim was not an experienced cook and, even though he was a good sport about things, I tried not to rely on him. That meant for many nights dinner was a salad mix and premade veggie burgers.

I abstained from sledding down Holmes Dam with my grandchildren because if we took a tumble, I wouldn't be able to catch myself without damaging my hands. Falling would mean landing on my face.

I also developed a strange fascination with people's hands. I would notice when someone was carrying a heavy load or playing with a child by swinging him or her in the air. I kept thinking how strong other people were and how amazing it was that they could perform the feats they did with their hands. Even watching TV, I found myself marveling at the actors' hand strength. I had to hold myself back from complimenting my friends constantly about how strong their hands were.

To my consternation, I realized that I could spend most of every day taking care of my hands. Unless carefully managed, a physical disability can become a social and emotional one. I didn't want to spend my life maintaining my health—I wanted to be fully alive and engaged with the world. I asked myself, "How much of my time should I spend doing things that are good for me? And how much time should I save to do things that are important to me?"

People were kind and helpful. The first lesson was how to accept help gracefully. The second lesson required learning not to accept any more help than necessary. It was all too easy to be waited on. I am fortunate to have a husband with a good sense of humor and loving friends. However, as time passed, I became more aware that this was my problem to deal with. Talking about my disability was not a conversation that cheered anyone up. Suggestions about what I should do were rarely helpful.

I needed to stay with my pain and grief until I could move on in a healthy manner. That winter I spent time meditating and also just watching the sky, the lake, and the birds flying overhead. I reminded myself of all the things I still could do: swim, read, talk, and walk outside.

Around this time several incidents changed my point of view. I went out to dinner with two friends and poured out my grief. My friend Cathy responded, "You have beautiful hands and you can still use them to talk. I have always loved to watch you talk with your hands." Jeanine added, "Your hands have served you well. They have worked long and hard for you and they have helped you build a good life. Remember to thank them for all the work they've done. Keep loving them."

Not long afterward, I watched the Leonid meteor showers. In less than an hour, I saw a grass-green shooting star unfurl slowly across the eastern sky, and dive-bomb into Holmes Lake. Many times during my life, when I have faced a significant hurdle, I've witnessed a green shooting star. This shooting star has been a reassuring signal from the universe.

The more I talked to my friends, the more I realized my suffering was nothing exceptional. My hand surgeon, who was a classical pianist, told me, "Your hands will get better, but they are always going to hurt.

You won't be seriously disabled and you'll always be able to do what you most need to do, but you will have pain. My hands hurt me every day too."

I thought about my grandmother the year after my grandfather died of a heart attack. She was dying of leukemia in her small home in Flagler, Colorado, and I visited her with my mother. When I asked about her health, my grandmother would say, "Let's talk about something more interesting." She would ask about my school, my reading, and my friends.

One day I told her that I greatly admired how she handled her difficult situation with such good cheer. She looked at me and said, "Mary, I have no choice about the leukemia, but I can control how I deal with it. I might as well act right and have something to feel good about."

While I had surgeries and rehabilitation, I heard that a friend's daughter was dying of liver cancer. I could hardly go to the library or gym without running into peers who had just lost someone or heard alarming health news about themselves. I realized that during my healthy days, I had taken so much for granted. My questions about my hands shifted from "Why me?" to "Why not me?"

When I first heard about my hands, I envisioned all the negative possibilities—decrepitude, dependency, and a gradual deterioration of all that truly mattered to me—but I realized the long view can be a perilous one to take. None of us knows what will happen in our futures, good or bad. It is much more adaptive to focus on building one good day at a time.

By springtime, I was more focused on appreciating what I could. I welcomed the earlier sunrises, the new green of the leaves, and my own awkward but healing body. Sometimes for a few minutes I could be in a state of deep gratitude.

One morning a cedar waxwing flew down to the grass beside me. I hadn't seen one of these birds in years, since a particularly cold spring had frozen our crabapple blossoms and many waxwings had starved beside our big tree. But here one was, a real beauty, migrating through and stopping by to say, "Nice to see you are outside today."

Now only when people ask me about my hands do I remember how badly damaged they are. They are better. I can use paperclips and scissors again. I am swimming more and gardening less. I am on my third version of dictation software. I have adapted.

As we age, we all experience "worn bodies." The luckiest suffer small losses and minor health issues. Others must face dire health emergencies. Most of us fall in between these two extremes. We work harder at being healthy and yet we experience more illnesses and pain. This life stage requires a constant process of adjustment and accommodation. We suffer a setback, we regain homeostasis, and soon we are enjoying our lives again.

We can help each other by talking and listening, by bringing the fruit plates or coffee cakes, and by writing loving notes. We can learn how to make everything workable. Our travails become crucible experiences that allow us to grow stronger and kinder. In spite of our grief, we can learn to find beauty. We understand the bittersweet nature of the universe, one of the most authentic and enlivening experiences possible.

CHAPTER 4

Intensity and Poignancy

"For the first time, I was pierced by the little panic and *tristesse*
occasioned by small things passing irrevocably from view."
—Faith Sullivan

"Today a red fox ran down through the corn stubble;
He vanished like smoke. I want to praise things
that cannot last." —Barbara Crooker

AT SIXTY-EIGHT, EMMA is a slender Irish redhead with freckles across her
nose and cheeks. She lives with her husband of forty-five years in Denver.
Chris runs a small landscaping business. The work is taking a toll on his
body but he keeps at it. Until her retirement three years ago, Emma was
a second-grade teacher.

Chris and Emma have three children—a son who lives in Florida,
another in Boulder, and a daughter named Alice, who lives a mile away

from them. All three have been married and divorced. The sons have remarried, but Alice has not. She depends on Chris and Emma for baby-sitting and financial help.

Just before school began, Emma invited over four of her grand-daughters, Alice's twins, age eight, and their nine- and ten-year-old cousins from Boulder. In the morning, while it was cool, they picked raspber-ries. When it heated up, they slipped indoors for a game of Clue. Then she drove them downtown for lunch at an outdoor café near Larimer Square. Emma challenged the girls to order one thing they had never before tasted. The twins ordered cucumber lemonades. The ten-year-old tried a lobster roll and her sister finished the meal with green tea ice cream.

Afterward the twins wanted to go to a bookstore. Emma agreed and offered to buy each girl one book. They browsed for over an hour. Emma showed them the books she'd loved as a girl and even read them a couple of poems. After the bookstore, they returned to Emma's for a swim in the neighborhood pool.

For Emma, it was a wonderful day. The girls made her laugh so hard her sides hurt. When they walked down the street, they still held her hand, but they had strong opinions about everything from waiters to how people should dress in a downtown café. Emma wasn't quite spiffy enough for their taste. They felt she should have worn nicer shoes.

From Emma's point of view, the girls were the perfect combination of smart and bold. She was delighted that they were more relaxed and free than she had been as a girl.

When Alice picked up all the girls at five o'clock, Emma was tired and ready for alone time. Still, as Alice drove away, she felt an aching in her heart. One of the twins had left her fidget spinner in the kitchen and, when Emma found it, she felt a pang of tenderness for the little things children possess.

Chris had a business meeting that night, so Emma fixed herself a PB and J and carried it to the balcony to watch the sun set over the mountains. She relived the joy of the day and laughed aloud when she remembered funny things the girls had said.

She also experienced a deep sense for how quickly time passes. Weren't these girls all newborns yesterday? And how could her own children be in their thirties and forties? Hadn't she been a girl herself only a short time ago? Wouldn't her lovely granddaughters be old women in the blink of an eye? These feelings swept over her like a rapidly moving cloud. She sighed at how precious life was and how ephemeral.

• • •

BY OUR SIXTIES, we may think the way we did in our forties, but our bodies don't act that age. Intimations of mortality can make us sad and fearful, but they can also wake us up. Until we understand how short life is, many of us make the mistake of thinking that our routines will go on forever. Our monthly book club, our Saturday card parties, or our Friday-night cocktails with friends feel as if they will never end. But after our awakening, we realize we've taken far too much for granted. We only have left a finite number of full moons, spring mornings, and nights out on the town. Families, friends, and country change and parts of our lives fade away.

And about the time we realize how many things are ending, time seems to speed up. At first, we think, "Where did today go?" then, "Where did this week go?" and finally, "Where did this year go?"

When I think of time now, I see an image from an old movie: pages of a calendar, each with a date on it, blow rapidly away as soon as they are turned by the wind.

We become aware that we may be doing some things for the last time. We visit our great aunt in her nineties. We bid goodbye to a friend who is moving to Florida. We complete the ten-mile hike up a mountain, but suspect we won't do it again. These last moments are poignant.

The English language contains the words "poignant" and "bitter-sweet," but it is challenging to find other words to describe the complex emotional states we feel as we run out of time. Our inner experience is too complicated to label.

Without language to express the nuances, we often resort to using single words to describe complicated feelings, but emotions frequently occur in combinations, such as sorrow and rage, anger and fear, or love, sadness, and bitterness all at the same time. We do not usually feel this or that, but rather, both this and that and three or four other emotions as well. I felt such a library of feelings when an old friend from Scotland visited us in the summer of 2016.

We first met Frank when he came to Nebraska in 1974 to partici-pate in a symposium at the university where my husband, Jim, and I were graduate students. We had offered to host a foreign visitor. Frank was scheduled to stay with us only three nights, but we enjoyed each other's company so much that he changed his ticket and stayed ten days. He was only ten years older than Jim and I were, but already he had written textbooks and was serving as president of the European Federation of Psychologists' Associations.

Frank had a much bigger grasp of world history, politics, and geog-raphy than we did. He held strong and well-reasoned opinions on everything—clinical psychology, governance in the U.K., capitalism, European politics, and the nature of the human race. He was fiercely proud of his country and his clan history. He knew a great deal about America's history and government and he expressed strong views about our country's role in the world.

When we met, Frank was a mountain climber and a member of a Scottish Mountain Rescue team. He had a thick Scottish accent, curly black hair, and a sturdy build. He always wore the same color slacks and shirt: blue and blue. For forty-two years, I've never seen him in any other outfit.

Frank is married to Frances, a psychologist like himself. Every other year we take turns "crossing the pond." We know Frank's children and grandchildren and they know ours. We regard each other as the Scottish and Nebraska branches of the same family.

Traditionally, we have hiked and backpacked in the Rocky Mountains and Scottish Highlands together. We have had uproarious times around campfires in wilderness areas and mountain meadows. One time I remember laughing so hard around a campfire that I said, "If we are not happy now, what on earth could make us happy?"

Now Frank is almost eighty and last year he had a stroke. When Frank got off the plane this year, he announced it was his farewell visit to Nebraska. As they walked toward us, Frances held his hand to steady him. The travel had been arduous and painful. Except for his walking and difficulty with balance, Frank was much the same. His intellect, sense of humor, and kindness remained intact.

On this trip there would be no hiking. However, we did many of our usual activities. For many nights in a row, we watched the moon rise over Holmes Lake. We savored long, slow meals and read together around our fireplace. We drank coffee in the mornings and talked, talked, talked about changes in our personal lives and the political landscape. We punctuated everything with laughter. Our conversations were those of people who had known each other for decades. We ranged freely across time and space and shared our emotions without hesitation.

Frank and I spoke about impending death. I read him Robert Frost's poem *Death of the Hired Man*. His favorite lines were, "Home is the place where, when you have to go there, / They have to take you in." In the same poem, home is also defined as "Something you somehow haven't to deserve." Both Frank and I find great comfort in poetry. Sometimes poetry is the only form of language that can express the complexity and depth of our emotions.

On the weekend, we watched my six-year-old grandson play soccer. Frank promised him tickets to a Manchester United game if he could come soon. Frances's brother works for Man U and she offered to send T-shirts and other team swag.

We visited my son's farm for a big meal. Frank told my son's three children about his experiences as a child in Scotland during the war. He recalled when his uncles were called to war and when one was killed. He had been a boy during the bombing and the starvation rations.

Frank became acquainted with our two-year-old grandson, Otis, who immediately loved Frank and held his hand when he needed a guide. He sat on his lap and even fed him from his own spoon. Frank dutifully ate whatever Otis put in his mouth, even though Otis clearly had a cold.

At one time, it seemed as if we would cross the pond and see each other forever. But now, forever was over. There was sadness—losing Frank would feel like losing a chunk of our being. But there was also sweetness—the sweetness of appreciating everything in the moment for just what it was.

The last morning, Frank told us that being with our five grandchildren made him optimistic that our good lives in Nebraska would continue far into the future. We watched the hummingbirds together one last time. We took every possible variety of group photo and then rode silently to the airport. Ordinary conversation seemed banal, and yet the truth was too complicated to voice.

At the airport, I gave Frank a book of collected poems by Robert Frost. He put it in his rucksack. We hugged goodbye in silence. From now on, any goodbye might well be the last.

Psychologist Laura Carstensen discovered that our perspectives and decisions change greatly depending on our perceptions of how much time we have left. The shorter we think our lives will be, the more likely we are to do things that are meaningful and give us pleasure. Awareness of death catapults us toward joy and reflection.

Carstensen found that with age we experience less anger and anxiety. I suspect that cannot be because we have less tragedy, but rather because we have better coping skills. Furthermore, knowing that our time is short, we tend to focus on joy. "Eventually" is no longer a word for us. We take our pleasures now.

When women receive a terminal diagnosis they often feel that they love being alive more than ever before. They find great enjoyment in their friends, family, and routines. When one local oncologist tells a patient that she has cancer, he says, "You are about to experience the most life-affirming era of your lifetime."

Of course, from birth on, our death is impending, but when it becomes imminent, we experience our lives on a deeper or profound emotional level. The great blessing that comes with a sense of finitude is gratitude. Many of us wake up every day feeling grateful to be alive. We enjoy the smallest of pleasures. Actually, there are no small pleasures. A cup of coffee with our neighbor, a song on the radio, or a walk with our dog can be exquisite.

We are more likely to tell people we love them and to hear that from them. We know that, any moment, we can change or they can change. Our hiking partner of today may be in a wheelchair tomorrow.

CHAPTER 5

Caregiving

"In all our contacts, it is probably the sense of being really
needed and wanted which gives us the greatest satisfaction
and creates the most lasting bond."
—Eleanor Roosevelt

CRYSTAL IS A trim Korean American woman who managed an ice-cream parlor until she retired. Once customers came in a couple of times, Crystal always remembered them. She and her husband, Joel, were my friends of the road. Jim and I dropped in for cones and we often attended the same concerts and worked together on community projects.

One Sunday, as I was looking over tomatoes at the farmers market, I saw Crystal pushing Joel in a wheelchair. Joel waved and smiled at me over the basket of produce he had in his lap. He conveyed his usual friendly persona, but his smile was crooked and his right arm hung by his side. I hugged him and we chatted for a minute. His speech was slower, softer, and more limited. Occasionally he scrambled words and I had to guess what he was trying to say. When he pointed to the bluegrass band nearby, Crystal rolled him over by the stage. Then she and I sat down under a cottonwood tree by the little creek that ran beside the market.

"After Joel's stroke, our lives became much smaller," she said. Joel suffered considerable cognitive impairment and required a great deal of physical therapy. Also, like many stroke patients, right after his stroke, he was depressed. Crystal said, "Joel's doing better now. At first, we were both overwhelmed. Overnight our lives morphed into something totally different."

Now Crystal's life is built around caring for Joel. She drives him to his appointments and helps him with his speech and physical therapy exercises. She pays the bills, deals with taxes, and, most frustrating of all, she manages all the insurance and medical and government paperwork. "You would not believe how many hours I spend examining manuals and bills," she said, shaking her head.

She misses the Joel who helped her work through ordinary human problems such as getting along with her siblings and dealing with a difficult neighbor. Joel had been empathic yet practical in his approach to relationship issues. He had known her family for decades and, at just the right moment, he could make a joke or suggestion. However, Joel still helps in any way he can. He is always there to listen and comfort Crystal. Sometimes he can't express his ideas the way he wants, but he can still joke, nod sympathetically, and put his good arm around her.

Crystal said that they are adjusting to their new lives. They listen to podcasts or watch comedies. Three times a week, she invites someone over for tea or drinks. Old friends come to visit and fill them in on what is going on around them.

"We don't compare our life now to our old life. It's a different life. But we still love each other and get along," Crystal continues. "I wouldn't want Joel anywhere but with me."

Crystal is a typical caregiver, a woman in our life stage caring for a family member with health problems. Her life has changed radically and she misses her former life, but she is making the best of her new situation.

Not all women who want to care for a family member can do it. Sometimes, they live a thousand miles away or have demanding jobs or health problems. Other times, they simply have too many people to care for and must make hard choices. Often women wish they could do more and feel guilty that they cannot.

Caregiving for most women can be immensely fulfilling and terribly difficult. It's the ultimate "both/and" experience. It provides us with the opportunity to feel useful but, at the same time, it can be isolating and hard on our health.

Traditionally, women have always cared for the old, the infirm, and the young. Like almost all generations before us, our generation of women was raised to be self-sacrificing. Our duties are not necessarily onerous. In fact, most of us have been caregivers all of our lives and continuing in this role can be satisfying. If we are lucky, we live in a rich web of interdependent relationships. We visit our friends in hospitals, make condolence casseroles, care for ill family members, and assist neighbors in times of need. We enjoy the people we help and know that some of them may later return the favor.

Caregiving requires us to put aside our own needs and sacrifice our time for the welfare of another. Especially as the work approaches full-time, it's bound to have its dismal aspects. Yet many people choose to do it and feel good about it. Because of its paradoxical nature, caregiving presents us an opportunity to explore the question "What do we mean by happiness?"

Caregiving provides many of us with meaning and purpose. In an era when 40 percent of Americans feel as if their lives have no meaning, this is no small benefit. Yet, a 2015 survey by the National Alliance for Caregiving found that almost 40 percent of caregivers find their work highly stressful and between 40 percent and 70 percent of caregivers suffer from depression.

In her essay "What is the Good Life?" Emily Esfahani Smith compares happy lives to meaningful ones. Happiness is about feeling good and getting what we want. In a sense, it is about taking. On the other hand, meaningful lives often involve suffering and self-sacrifice in the service of a transcendent purpose. However, Smith concludes, "Happiness seekers are unhappy when they don't get what they want. Meaning seekers can survive negative events."

The question here is, how do we define happiness? We don't have adequate words to parse its many forms, and we could benefit from more nuanced language. We need a word for the happiness we feel eating ice cream at a festival, after making love on a lazy fall afternoon, on hearing that one of our grandchildren won a scholarship, or when we run into a long-lost friend at an airport.

Contentment is a form of happiness, as is excitement over interesting things happening. Anticipating a vacation or a Saturday-night party is one kind of happiness, and getting a good night's sleep and waking up refreshed is another. Finally, there is the happiness that comes from helping other people and doing our duty. We need all these kinds of happiness in some particular balance. It's the balance that is tricky.

American culture doesn't make it easy to sort through this issue. Americans tend to value work that produces income, but actually, the most important work for society often doesn't do that. Sadly, professional caregivers are poorly paid and many unpaid caregivers are not acknowledged for their constant efforts. If we define work as the creation of the good on earth, then caregiving is some of the best work we can do.

As friends or family members and caregivers, we can help a great deal by listening and empathizing with women who are in the thick of it. We can bring them small gifts, such as books, chocolates, or flowers, and make sure they are invited to get-togethers even if it is unlikely they will make it. When women are homebound caretakers, a daily phone call can be a lifesaver. We can acknowledge both the efforts other women are making and validate the importance of those efforts.

Ardith is a graphic artist who takes care of a cantankerous mother. Her mother should be in a care facility, but refuses to go. Several times a day, she calls Ardith demanding that she come fix her garbage disposal, help her with her hair, or wash her clothes. When Ardith does these things, her mother doesn't thank her. She takes it for granted that Ardith will serve her in all ways.

While Ardith does her best to set limits, she does not want her mother to suffer. That means that, after long days of work, she drives to her mother's instead of going home to cook a meal for herself and her husband. Ardith is tired all the time and sighs whenever she speaks of her mother.

Over time, her relationship with her mother has affected her marriage and her mental health. She knows her husband will stay loyal, but she feels guilty that she misses so much time with him. She cannot help but feel used and bitter. Ardith told me, "I received awards for my art, but nothing for Mom Duty."

"I'm buying you a trophy and a dozen roses," I said.

Ardith laughed and said, "Just buy me the roses. Yellow, please."

I bought the roses but, at the same time, I know that Ardith's and all other caregivers' primary validation must be internal. When we do something arduous such as deal with an insurance company all day, we must give ourselves credit for our skill and persistence. At the end of a difficult afternoon, we need to remind ourselves that we perform honorable labor and that there will be better days. That is harder than it sounds. Perhaps caregivers should tape a note on their bathroom mirrors reminding them to praise themselves for their day's labors.

As Ardith told me, "Nothing I've ever done is as punishing as caring for my mother. I have no time for myself. I oscillate between guilt and rage. My blood pressure is up."

She continued. "I tell myself I am earning stars in my crown for heaven. On my deathbed, this will be what I am most proud of. I persevered at a thankless task simply because it was the right thing to do."

When we are caring for anyone on a full-time basis, we must learn to balance taking care of others with taking care of ourselves. We need to develop a truly effective self-care plan. Step one of our plan can be exploring and accepting our own emotions about the situation. We can acknowledge our ambivalence, our anger, frustration, and bitterness. We can go outside and scream in frustration or break down and cry for as long as we need to. Expressing strong emotions is actually a skillful way to relieve them.

We may need to set more limits. Ardith, for example, may sometimes need to say no to her crabby, ungrateful mom. But setting limits with sick loved ones usually necessitates considerable retraining. We women are socialized to feel responsible for everyone and, if we aren't careful, we can have so much empathy that we wear ourselves down meeting others' needs.

When we sense this is happening, it's important to refocus on what we must do for ourselves in order to stay vital. This could be meditation, taking our dog for a walk, dinner out, sleeping in, or working in our garden. Once we know what we need, then we can explain to others that we will be there to help after we have cared for ourselves. Then, instead of feeling guilty, we can praise ourselves for setting healthy limits. This kind of self-protection is especially important when we are caring for someone who may need us for a long time.

We may want to ask for help from friends and family members or find a support group and schedule days off for self-care. If the person we are caring for is homebound, we can invite in visitors. A home with people coming and going is cheerful and can help our loved one keep up on the news.

• • •

WILLOW'S HUSBAND, SAUL, had trouble with balance and had fallen twice on the way to his bookstore. Willow suspected he had some kind of ear infection. She encouraged him to see his doctor and, one afternoon, Saul closed his bookstore and went in for a checkup. The doctor ordered tests and asked Saul to come in for results in a month. Willow wanted to go with him, but she was writing a grant. Saul was alone when he heard that he had mid-stage Parkinson's and was likely to soon have more serious symptoms.

At dinner, in his low-key way, Saul told Willow about his diagnosis and prognosis. Willow pushed away her plate and sobbed. Saul patted her arm and murmured, "We'll be okay. Let me worry about this."

In addition to her sorrow, Willow was frightened that Saul's health eventually would interfere with her career, but he didn't ask her to make any changes. However, that next month, Saul put the bookstore up for sale and hired someone to manage it until it sold.

For a while, things went on as normal. Saul flew alone to visit his brother in California. He joined an exercise group for Parkinson's patients and continued to see friends and visit bookstores. But a year later, he fell and broke his wrist. He needed Willow's help to dress and shower. His tremors worsened and, when he was tired, his head rolled from side to side. He had a hard time making eye contact.

At first, Willow felt overwhelmed. Her life had been upended and many of her assumptions about the future no longer held. Resources for Saul were not in place and everything required new learning. Despite her career working with people in need, Willow felt totally unprepared to be a caregiver in her personal life.

After dinner one night, Willow blurted out, "Retirement makes me think of being isolated, tired, and lying around all day in pajamas doing nothing."

"We'd be together," Saul replied. "Can't you imagine that being fun?"

Willow honestly could not. She worried about her clients Ruby and Myron and all the others she would be abandoning. She wondered if she and Saul would get on each other's nerves or become one of those couples with nothing to say to each other. When she pictured a life of putting on Saul's shoes or helping him to the bathroom, it looked so dismal.

As they waited for a cab one evening, Willow repeated her worries about retirement. Saul looked at her with exasperated tenderness and said, "If I ever need help at home, we will hire a caregiver. The most important thing is that you be happy."

Willow was reassured by this comment, but it made her feel guilty. Meanwhile she kept working, but she left the office at five so that she could make it home in time for Saul's physical therapy. This arrangement wasn't ideal for either of them. She rushed out before her day's work was done and Saul was alone all day.

Willow felt exhausted and unfocused. Saul had been the one who had cooked and cared for her. She knew she had emotionally difficult decisions ahead. She wanted to do the right thing for Saul, but she loved running the show at work, and all of a sudden, her show was in its third act.

At home, she had times when she snapped at Saul or wondered if she was courageous enough for the fate she was facing. She prayed for strength.

Yet, at the same time, emergencies called for emergent behavior. Not everyone experiences growth when growth is required, but Willow slowly grew into a better version of herself. She accepted the new reality and switched from seeing herself as a victim to seeing herself as a volunteer.

Over the next year, as Saul's health deteriorated, Willow became stronger by simply meeting each new challenge. Day after day she helped Saul with his many physical needs, and slowly she acquired more patience and endurance. She developed a strong set of internal resources, and she grew into a more empathic woman. Her relationship with Saul became both deeper and more fun.

Willow continued to balance work and care for Saul. She was determined to make both their time and her time enjoyable and, mostly, she succeeded. She had been a good coper all of her life and she was resilient now.

She knew that when Mother Teresa was dying, she said, "I have worked for God all of my life and I know I will soon be dancing in heaven. But I wish I had danced more during my time on earth." No matter what situation she was in, Willow was determined to find some moments for dancing.

CHAPTER 6

Swept Away

"Down, down, down into the darkness of the grave
Gently they go, the beautiful, the tender, the kind;
Quietly they go, the intelligent, the witty, the brave.
I know. But I do not approve. And I am not
resigned." —Edna St. Vincent Millay

"Life was meant to be lived, and curiosity must be kept alive.
One must never, for whatever reason, turn his back on life."
—Eleanor Roosevelt

JENNY'S PARENTS LIVED three hours away in a small Nebraska town. The last year of their lives, Jenny drove out to see them once a week and chauffeured them to doctors' appointments. In between visits, she texted them multiple times a day and Skyped with them every evening. Caring for her parents felt like a full-time job, but Jenny did not complain. Rather, she saw the whole year as her last chance to be connected to them.

The weekend before her mother died, she told Jenny that she was ready to go. She was tired of all of her ailments and no longer enjoyed her life. Jenny organized that last weekend so that her mother was with her children and grandchildren. Her mother was comfortable, alert, and able to laugh and talk in ways that left all of her family with good memories. After the rest of the family left, Jenny stayed with her. On Tuesday night, her mom died in her sleep.

Jenny brought her father, who used a wheelchair, home to live with her family. She fixed his favorite foods and her son played piano for him. They watched old movies and played cribbage. A month later, he, too, died.

The funeral was held in the small-town church her parents had attended for almost sixty years. Jenny told those gathered not to mourn because her parents "had good lives." At the reception afterward, Jenny told me, "Being with my parents while they died was the most difficult and beautiful experience of my life."

Jenny missed them, but her grief was not intense. Because her parents had lived a long time, and because she had been able to care for them, Jenny found it relatively easy to say goodbye.

Helping someone die is an honor and a responsibility. It changes us. However unwillingly, we learn lessons about the nature of reality and about ourselves. Of course, we are not always able to help. Death can be sudden and unexpected. We may be far away and have many demands on our time. Sometimes, in spite of our best efforts, the process of dying can be deeply miserable. But if we are lucky, we have some time and some agency.

Next to birth, death is the most elemental and mysterious of human experiences. But, unlike birth, where we have a reasonable sense of what happens next, with death everything is shrouded in mystery.

Death is a social, emotional, spiritual, and physical event. It is also a culturally scripted one. Our American culture is in denial about death. We are not encouraged to discuss it or contemplate it. Often when we try to talk about it we are told, "Don't be morbid." We are not educated about how to communicate with dying loved ones about their approaching deaths. Because of this, we sometimes miss opportunities for saying what should be said and holding healing conversations. We often experience on-the-job training.

If we are helping another person face death, we want to make sure we are clear about their wishes around death and dying. If we are fortunate, they will stay alert and will be able to make their own decisions. If we must be *deciders*, we want to have as much information of our loved ones' wishes as possible.

It is important to have in place medical powers of attorney, end-of-life directives, instructions on funeral wishes, a will, but perhaps most important, we need a family understanding about end-of-life care. This involves not one conversation, but many conversations over the years with all relevant relatives. Many Americans wait until the last minute to have these talks, but a crisis is not the ideal time to discuss complicated, intense life choices.

Hospice can be of great help to us. With few exceptions, its workers are skilled at treating physical, emotional, and spiritual pain. Hospice encourages patients to accept death and the experiences that dying brings. When people are dying, they are often scared of pain, scared of the process of dying, and scared of being helpless and alone. Often, they have practical problems with breathing, eating, digestion, and mobility. Hospice can help people die with dignity.

Rosalee, a hospice worker, told me that often the agony that people feel around death is not from physical pain, which can usually be controlled, but rather from emotional pain and fear for the future. She gave the example of a man dying of throat cancer. He had abandoned his family when the children were young and now he felt guilty and ashamed of his earlier behavior. He wished his sons were there so he could apologize, but they were not speaking to him. She also told me about a woman who was terrified she would lose her cognitive capacities before she died and become someone who was crude and out of control.

"We can't fix everything," Rosalee said. "Sometimes we just hold hands and listen."

She said that when families try to keep dying relatives from knowing about their medical situation, death is more difficult. Most of the time, people know and yearn for their family to face it with them. Hospice teaches that there are five essential conversations: "Please forgive me. I forgive you. I love you. Thank you. Goodbye."

"In hospice, women tend to live longer than men," Rosalee said. "Women have an easier time with emotional conversations and they are more likely to accept more alternative therapies such as massage and aromatherapy."

Sometimes, hospice patients appreciated jokes or stories about life outside the room. Many appreciated being touched or having their hair combed or lotion applied. Rosalee often gave people foot and head massages. She knew to ask, "What joy can I make happen today? In the next five minutes? Right now?"

Rosalee advised that we don't want to enter a hospice patient's room with an agenda. We don't want to discuss our troubles or offer false reassurances. Also, most dying people do not enjoy hearing about other people who are dying or who have their same health problems. They would rather talk about happy times in the past or positive events in the present. Most people appreciate knowing that they have mattered and that they have been kind and thoughtful people.

Rosalee also observed that while in our culture we emphasize being with our loved ones when they die, many people wait to die until their family leaves the room. She speculated that this is because it is hard to let go of life surrounded by family. It is easier to let go when alone by simply drifting away.

Rosalie said that most of us want the same things when we die. We want to be at home, with family or close friends, comfortable, and clearheaded.

Unlike hospice, our modern medical system encourages us to deny death. Even in cases of terminal cancer, doctors are inclined to offer more treatments. As Dr. Atul Gawande wrote in *Being Mortal: Medicine and What Matters in the End*, "Doctors are not trained to help their patients make good decisions about how to manage fatal diseases. Rather, they are trained to save lives and encourage hope. So, they recommend procedures they would not accept for themselves."

As Dr. Gawande writes, many doctors do not want the late-stage treatments they prescribe. In his research, a study headed by V. J. Periyakoil found that 88 percent of physicians said they would avoid invasive procedures and life-prolonging machines as they approached the end of their lives.

Mavis helped her husband die a good death. She drove Rick to a doctor's appointment for a biopsy on June 1. On June 5, they heard he had liver cancer that had spread through his body. The doctor recommended some palliative treatments that would require him to stay in the hospital, but Rick wanted to go home. Mavis picked up the phone and ordered a hospital bed for their apartment. She checked into hospice services and, later that day, she drove Rick home.

Her focus was totally on Rick. She wanted to meet his needs, organize his medical care, and help him feel comfortable, loved, and happy. She fixed his favorite chicken noodle soup and bought fresh fruit for smoothies. She found a massage therapist who would make house calls. Mavis got in touch with everyone who had tangled with Rick and asked them to visit and resolve their issues with him. She asked friends, co-workers, and relatives to write notes and letters about what he meant to them.

A hospice worker made sure Mavis had the necessary pain medications and equipment for Rick and taught her how to give him injections. Mavis bucked up and was the best version of herself. She had no idea she was capable of so much competent and loving action.

For the next month, Rick was home and, with the help of hospice, didn't suffer physically. On the Fourth of July, they watched the fireworks over a nearby city park a few blocks away. They toasted their happy marriage with champagne. Rick had only a few sips. Mavis held his hand, watched the exploding sky, and finished the bottle. The next day, when Rick died, Mavis was cradling him in her arms. She had given him the death that he wanted.

Mavis gained strength through her experiences. Rick had always taken care of her. He had handled most of the practical details of their lives. Caring for him allowed her to be the strong one. She felt she had repaid him for some of his loving care of her. After Rick's death, Mavis cried for six hours. Then she called a few friends and relatives. Three days later, Rick was cremated, and his ashes were buried in a nearby cemetery.

Afterward the house felt so empty. When workers removed the hospital bed from her living room, it felt as if she didn't have enough furniture. She had been so focused on Rick that when he died, there was nothing left inside her. Grief moved into all of the spaces in her heart.

Indeed, her whole body seemed in shock. She felt numb and unable to move. She could hardly think, speak, or breathe. All around her was a deep darkness that signified a loss of all hope. She kept thinking, "I wish I could go with him."

She didn't believe in suicide because of the damage to friends and family members left behind, but she wanted to be dead. She felt as if she would never be happy again. Her life seemed over.

Three years later, while Mavis still felt lonely, she had learned some things. She had learned to ask for support from her own friends and family. When she walked into her church or pottery class, she said, "I need hugs. I need to be love-bombed."

She understood how to help others who had lost family members. Never again would she say, "Let me know if there's anything I can do."

Instead, she would take over a meal, invite the bereaved to a movie, or set up a regular time for coffee.

She also learned how to take things a day at a time. When she looked far into the future she was overwhelmed by all the possibilities. But when she focused on making it through each day in the best way possible, she could often meet her goal. Her most important lesson was that she was stronger and kinder than she realized.

My nephew Paul guides young people into the California wilderness for several weeks at a time. He told me, "While we are out, I want a big storm to come up. I want hard, cold rain to fall and wind to blow the tents down. That is when the kids find out what they are made of."

Losing a loved one is rather like being in a bad storm. We find out things about ourselves. Often, we discover surprising reserves of strength and courage.

There is a big difference between helping loved ones die and losing them. When we are helping, we have focus and meaning. Our loved one is still with us. When they die, we are often adrift and empty. As one friend put it, "I feel as if I am half of something that no longer exists."

Sudden deaths, untimely deaths, such as the death of a child, and deaths that could have been prevented are the heaviest to bear. However, even when we are expecting them, all deaths feel sudden. A person is inspirited in one minute and in the next minute she is a corpse.

Our shock is followed by a dark sense that nothing will be workable.

We are in a crucible moment where all of our reserves will be tested. We have lost sight of one shore, but cannot yet see the other.

Grief is a physical and emotional experience. It's important to actually feel our own pain and to allow it time to unfurl. At first, we are so lonely. When we wake in the morning, our first thought is of our loss, and the day darkens. We want comfort in our grief from the very person we have lost. We can hardly face eating meals alone or our first few Saturday nights.

Yet, most of us progress though our grief. Often, we see how many people love us. Friends who know what bereavement feels like help us through the recovery process. We pass through all the expected stages of grief, but we also face what psychologist John Bowlby posits as an additional stage of grief, "yearning and searching." He describes this experience as a deep feeling of emptiness and a yearning to be with the loved one. The grieving often includes seeing our departed loved ones, talking to them, and feeling their presence.

Many of the women I spoke with described this yearning and searching. Sharon walked alone under the stars. When she was in a particular spot on her walk, she would look for a shooting star. She felt her husband beside her, protecting her. Three years after his death, she continued to see "his" falling stars.

True grief never goes away. We learn to live with it. After a while, our friends stop asking and we stop discussing our sorrows. It doesn't help us that much and we realize that almost everyone who we have confided in carries grief deep in their hearts too. We often decide that, once again, our job is to cheer others up.

Grief isn't just something to endure; it also is a reflection of our capacity to love. It allows us to understand the most profound human experience at the most intimate level. Facing our grief requires openness and courage. We must explore it with curiosity and patience and we must allow it to stay in our hearts until it is ready to leave.

Over time, by simply abiding with our sorrows, they will lessen. Yet, as poet Linda Pastan wrote, "Grief is a circular staircase." We feel better, and then we feel worse. Holidays, anniversaries, and many other things trigger grief reactions. We may have a rather good Year Two and then be felled by Year Three. With intention and skills, we move forward on our journey, but not without spiraling in the waters.

Eventually we will learn to rebalance our lives and achieve some separation from our grief. We don't want to drown in our grief or to be utterly detached from it. But, in the beginning, we can't know how to do this. Even eating dark chocolate, our hearts crack open with sorrow.

When we lose loved ones, we must search for our resilient self who knows how to proceed. That self will not appear immediately, but she lives deep within us waiting to be helpful.

We can remember our role models for healing. I called my eighty-year-old Aunt Grace after her son died of a heart attack. She lived in the Ozarks, surrounded by family. I was in Seattle on a book tour, but I wanted to be with my aunt so badly that my heart physically hurt. When she picked up the phone, I poured out my sorrow. Aunt Grace listened to me and reassured me that she felt my sympathy. Then she told me, "We just have to love and take care of the ones who are left."

Whenever I lose someone I remember Aunt Grace. No matter what our situation, we always have the existential freedom to make choices. There is always the opportunity for reflection and redemption.

Pat is a good example of a woman who faced her grief fully, made good choices, and spoke of her experience with wisdom and honesty. Pat's husband died two years ago. I had gone to his funeral. Jerry died at fifty-seven, but he had more good days than most people who live to be one hundred. Over the years he ran a food co-op, taught philosophy, and worked for Nebraska's public radio network. He loved his wife, his cats, good conversation, baseball, and playing the accordion. A William Stafford poem begins with this line: "When they shook the box and poured out its chances, you were appointed to be happy." Jerry was happy.

Recently Pat and I sat in her bright kitchen and discussed the time when Jerry was dying and its aftermath. She said that his esophageal cancer was a big surprise. Jerry and Pat had gone to Jerry's doctor for what they thought would be a routine endoscopy. Instead, the doctor immediately told them, "I see cancer." He scheduled Jerry for a CT scan the next day and, after that, his doctor told them that Jerry had no more than a year to live. Pat remembers that her first thought was, "We won't grow old together."

"Everything happened so fast. We first saw the doctor on December thirteenth. On December twentieth, we heard the cancer had spread to his liver and other organs. We told our family before Christmas and, after he started his treatment in early January, we told our friends. We planned for a year together."

Pat said that during that time she felt as if an alarm clock was always ringing in her brain, signaling a sense of urgency about what she needed to do next to help Jerry.

"I thought Jerry would be sick but that he would be the same Jerry. But I learned quickly that when someone is terribly sick they change," she explained. "I expected that we would take care of each other through this, but it became clear that our lives needed to be all about Jerry." She gave a small but telling example from the trip to Texas they took at Christmas to see his parents. Jerry had always handled the tickets and managed the details of flying, but this time, as soon as they walked into the airport, he handed Pat the tickets and depended on her to navigate.

During most of January Pat kept working at her job as director of a large city library system. She thought she would need her time off later when Jerry really was dying. Neither one of them realized he was dying that month.

When Pat was with Jerry she was busy. But on her way to work, she would be flooded by her dark thoughts. One of them was that her happiest days were behind her. The other was that she would either have to be alone or eventually date someone. When she said the phrase "date someone" to herself, she shuddered.

Pat recalled how Jerry described the cancer: "It felt as if I had been walking down the street and a giant came out of nowhere and threw me to the ground. I struggled but I couldn't get up."

Doctors had told Jerry he must eat and keep weight on, but eventually he could not make himself eat. He was upset that he didn't have the willpower to do that. People brought lovely food for him, custard and consommé, but he could not hold anything down. Because both his lungs and liver were failing, he endured many unpleasant symptoms, including hiccups and nonstop vomiting. Jerry was not afraid of death but he hated being so sick.

In late January, he went into the hospital on a Monday for what they hoped would be a quick stay before he returned home in better shape. Instead, they were told that it was time for palliative care and that Jerry had less than a month to live. Pat said she focused on getting their home ready for Jerry, and Jerry ready to go home. But Jerry never made it home; he died on Friday at the hospital.

Pat regretted that even though the doctor said she could bring their cats to visit Jerry in the hospital, she was too overwhelmed to do it. "Jerry loved those cats," she said.

Her parents and both of their extended families came to say goodbye. Pat's main goal for Jerry was that he would die feeling loved and surrounded by family, and she was able to give him that.

During the intense time when Jerry was rapidly dying, Pat felt great clarity about what was and wasn't essential in life. She learned quickly that some things were much more important than others, and that the most important thing was just being present for Jerry.

Jerry wasn't a churchgoer, but his funeral was held at Pat's church. He was a big supporter of the local chamber music quartet, and they provided beautiful music. More than six hundred people filled the church and it was standing room only inside and out. Jerry's parents from Texas were surprised by how many friends he had. They had not realized what an impact he had had on so many people. I was surprised too. I thought he and I had a special relationship and then realized that Jerry probably had a special relationship with all those other people too.

Afterward we all ate pie and sipped coffee in the basement of the church. Pat acted her usual self, poised and laughing with people. One of her relatives who had been at the hospital whispered to me, "If I ever have a fatal disease, I am calling Pat to take charge. I couldn't believe how efficient and organized she was at getting Jerry's needs met."

Now, two years later, as we reflected on the time since Jerry had passed, Pat expressed satisfaction at their years together. She and Jerry always had a good relationship with minimal tension and plenty of fun. Neither of them felt that they had wasted time not appreciating each other. She expressed surprise that since Jerry's death, she never had experienced a sobbing session. However, she had felt enfeebled and vulnerable, too weak to lift what seemed like a backpack full of pain. Fortunately, her friends and family gathered around her to help her to right the backpack and put it on her shoulders. She said, "Sometimes people even carried it for a while."

She described the first year after Jerry's death as mournful. The second year she called her grumpy year. She was full of outrage that a good person like Jerry had died so young. But she quoted Jerry himself on the topic, "Thinking that because you're a good person, bad things will not happen to you is like thinking that because you're a vegetarian, a bull won't charge you."

People would ask her how she was coping so well. She thought to herself, "What's my choice? I had to go to work to pay the bills. I didn't want to just lie around on my couch and do nothing. This is my world now; I'll deal with it."

Two years later Pat is not reconciled to her loss. She said, "I liked being married to Jerry." She smiled as she told me what she missed the most. Jerry was good at imitating sounds. If a board flapped in the wind or a pipe groaned, he would immediately make that exact sound. To this day, whenever she hears a sound around the house, she waits in vain for its echo.

Pat has plenty of friends and events to fill her days. At work, she has constant opportunities to grow and learn. But she still doesn't like coming home to an empty house.

Pat doesn't believe that everything happens for a reason. She sees Jerry's cancer as part of the randomness of the universe. However, she has tried to learn from it and to help others. She joined a Facebook group for people coping with esophageal cancer. She takes comfort in being useful.

Pat's mantra is "It's good to be alive." Jerry was always telling her to be present, and she tries to honor Jerry by noticing every good moment. "Joy is my best tribute to his memory."

Pat's story illustrates the complexity and longevity of grief. In one sense grief never ends. Yet it can be ameliorated. It helps to stay busy. It helps to have some form of creative expression. And it helps to have relationships. Pat is a resilient and competent person deeply embedded in a stable, supportive community. But she has not stopped hurting.

It is often said that the first year of widowhood is the hardest and then things improve, but in my experience with friends, the second year is often harder. This is partly because women have the expectation that after the first year they will feel better, and then they don't. This causes them to wonder what is wrong with them and to feel hopeless about recovering from grief.

Our culture has a short attention span and does not expect us to mourn anything for long, but the heart has a different timeline. As songwriter Mary Gauthier wrote, "A year is a drop in a bucket when you lose someone you love."

One of the best and worst things about life is that it goes on. For women who make good choices and develop good navigational skills, the tincture of time will facilitate recovery.

Many of us have rituals to help us heal. I find comfort in writing private eulogies where I explore what the person meant to me, why their life mattered, and what was truly unique about them. I also try to remember one great moment we had together.

Often, we associate departed family members with certain symbols. Many women find comfort and connection to their loved ones in birds, especially cardinals. A surprising number of women have told me stories of a cardinal showing up to sing to them after they lost a loved one. We also associate music, foods, places, and natural phenomena, such as the moon or shooting stars, with our departed loved ones. Whenever I catch a fish, I think of my father who loved all kinds of fishing. As my way to greet him, I hold my fish up to the sky.

Loss reminds us to wake up and to cherish. It pushes us to seek out beauty and love. We search for a transcendent response that helps us balance our suffering with meaning. Transcendent responses shine all around us—the memorial benches on a walking trail, the trees planted in someone's honor, and the financial donations to good causes. Even the simple act of putting flowers on a grave site can be a moment of transcendence. For us to survive loss, we must grow, and it is this growth that will propel us into a life of even greater meaning and gratitude.

CHAPTER 7

Loneliness and Solitude

"Life may be brimming over with experiences, but somewhere, deep inside, all of us carry a vast and fruitful loneliness wherever we go." —Etty Hillesum

CARLA HAD BEEN a fixture in my life for more than forty years. She was married to a musician and was part of our community of musicians and their fans. I saw her at parties, art openings, and fundraisers for nonprofits. She was always surrounded by friends. However, one evening at an outdoor concert, she told me she was lonely.

"It's ordinary loneliness," she said. "My husband is an introvert, our kids are gone, and I can spend days at home working on projects without seeing anyone."

"I can be lonely too," I said. "For almost exactly the same reasons. I spend a great deal of my life reading or writing. I am choosing this life, but it leaves me isolated."

We talked about how as we age we spend less time with others. We reminisced about the good old days when we called our friends for conversation whenever we wanted to talk. We text or email these days, and it feels intrusive, almost rude, to just call a friend out of the blue.

Carla sighed and said, "I like my life, but our house is so quiet. Sometimes I yearn for the years when I woke up with children, worked full-time in a busy clinic, made a quick family meal, and headed out with a carload of kids for soccer games or marching band practice."

No matter how we structure our lives, most of us will spend more time alone as we grow older. Data scientist Henrik Lindberg discovered that between ages twenty and forty, adults spend less than four hours a day alone. At seventy, the average person spends about seven hours a day alone. Whether that alone time is labeled as loneliness or solitude depends on our attitudes toward it and what we do with it. We older women are likely to experience a mix of loneliness and solitude.

Of course, we can feel alone all across our life spans. Childhood can be incredibly lonely, especially without emotionally available parents and a loving community. Children can be bullied and lonely at school, and teenagers tend to feel everything intensely, including loneliness. Stay-at-home moms can be isolated. Loneliness isn't unique to our age group but, because of the nature of this developmental stage, it's more inevitable.

Most of us have experienced losses by the time we turn sixty-five. We may outlive some of the people who loved us. We may retire and lose work colleagues or have mobility issues, hearing loss, or poor eyesight that limits our interactions with others. We may no longer drive. Our lack of good public transportation, poverty, or fear of crime may keep us more homebound than we would wish. Depression, low energy, or chronic illness can keep us from making and keeping friends.

Other people's decisions can have great effects on our lives. Holly had never married, but she hadn't been lonely. She had raised a daughter, Mandy, who had married and bought a house a block away. Over the years Mandy and her husband, Dave, had five children. Holly was present at their births and later watched the children while their parents worked. She attended all the children's events and it felt to her like they were one family in two houses.

One March day, when the oldest girl was ten and the baby was two, Mandy called with some startling news. Dave was being transferred to a city 1,000 miles away. The family would be moving when the school year ended. Mandy hadn't told her this might happen because she didn't want to upset her until they knew for sure, but just that morning Dave had received a call from his boss.

Holly was sitting in her old recliner when she heard the news. At first, she couldn't absorb it at all. Then she felt a great pressure on her chest and couldn't breathe. She thought she was having a heart attack. A few minutes later, when the pain subsided, Holly thought, "I may live through this, but I don't want to. I cannot go through this pain again."

When Holly was nine, her mother died of breast cancer and Holly was left with a bereft, emotionally distant father. She remembered that dark, hard time on a visceral level. Until Mandy was born, Holly had lived in darkness. Then, for the first time since she was nine, Holly had someone to love. These last few years, Mandy's big, exuberant family had given her the sunshine she needed. Now the darkness was returning.

An hour later, Mandy called back and offered to come by. Holly said no; she couldn't bear to let Mandy see her this broken. Instead she sat inside, staring out the window at the mud and dirty snow. "The children . . ." she thought. "How can I live without the children?"

She considered moving with them, and maybe she would. But she didn't have much money and doubted she could find a place she could afford in the new city. Besides, her church, friends of a lifetime, and mother's grave were all here.

Later, when she finally stood up, she poured a big glass of vodka from the bottle she kept in the freezer for company. She didn't often drink, but now seemed like a good time to anesthetize herself. She took a big gulp, choked, and then she sipped a little more. She didn't like the taste, and she could tell it wouldn't help anyway. This wasn't the kind of pain she could obliterate with booze.

Holly thought of two-year-old Freddy, of the way he felt in the curve of her body and of his soft hair that smelled of baby shampoo. With FaceTime she couldn't cuddle her grandson or smell his sweet aroma. She again had trouble breathing. She said to herself, "I can't bear it. I simply can't bear it."

People don't need to die for us to experience loss. Holly was losing her local family to a move. It felt to her as if there would be a death. In the 1800s, the Irish had emigration wakes for their families when they moved to America, never to return. They spoke elegies for the living. Holly felt elegiac now. Everything seemed so over.

Of course, Holly would visit and the family would come stay with her. In between visits, she would FaceTime the grandchildren. However, a year later, Holly still misses that family. Even though she is back in her comforting routines, she will carry her grief forever.

Joyce was also affected by other people's decisions. She had a life-long habit of going to the casino with her friend Annie from work. But Annie moved away. Joyce kept going to the casino on her own but it wasn't the same, and after her retirement, on her small fixed income, she could no longer afford nights at the casino. She spent her time playing Sudoku and watching television. She called herself a loner, but really, she was just alone. As she did housework, she held conversations with herself.

Two Thanksgivings ago, my friend Sandra's daughter had called her a bitch and stomped out the door after the meal. Sandra couldn't figure out why. She had mentioned that the fresh turkey was expensive and that she'd bought a $20 bottle of wine for the table, but that wouldn't normally upset Emily.

The two had a relationship full of conflict, but to Sandra's knowledge, nothing special had happened to make things worse. Sandra eventually decided Emily's behavior wasn't personal. She knew that Emily and her husband had recently refinanced their house and that they had credit card debt. Perhaps that was what made Emily extra insecure and defensive.

After that Thanksgiving, Emily avoided her. At one point, Sandra wrote a letter and asked if the two of them could discuss whatever was happening. Emily responded that she wanted to terminate the relationship. Sandra was floored. This seemed like a nightmare to her. How could this have happened?

She called and asked her daughter's husband what went wrong. He was sympathetic to her but said that Emily would need to speak for herself. Sandra's friends were sympathetic, but what could they do?

Sandra was angry. She had done her best with Emily. It wasn't her fault that, when Emily was three, her husband left them and moved in with his girlfriend. Later, Sandra worked double shifts so that Emily could be on the swim team and have nice clothes. She'd even paid for Emily's therapy when she was a teenager. Emily had been difficult, yet Sandra missed her. On her birthday and Mother's Day, she cried and cried. Twice she had written Emily and once she had called. Sandra kept busy, but she longed to talk to her daughter. She thought, "If only I could see her we could work things out." She felt bereft. What a tragedy.

Some women find themselves lonely later in life because they haven't valued relationships enough to cultivate them. Instead they've prioritized work or travel. This strategy may work when they are young, but can become harder when they are old. Recently I visited Mona in Santa Monica. She worked from home as a marketing consultant. Her garden was full of flowers, including her specialty, exotic orchids. She was a sophisticated woman with all kinds of resources, but she was lonely.

Over limeades in the garden, Mona told me she had been too busy to form friendships. Her only long-term relationships had been with her clients. She had succeeded in an expensive city by working ten hours a day. Now she wished she had some women friends.

At five every morning, she attended Pilates, but she had never asked any of her classmates out for coffee. Like her, they were on their way to work. Instead, she drove home, made some coffee, and fired up her laptop.

Almost all of her social time now came from social media. She posted mostly about her garden, fashion, and home design. Every evening she poured herself a gin and tonic and caught up with her online communications. "That isn't enough anymore," said Mona. "I want hugs and someone to talk to."

I asked her about prospects for local friends. Mona swallowed hard and looked out on her garden. "There is one woman in my Pilates class that I might ask out for coffee."

I told her I hoped she would do that. Mona was coming late to her realization that friendships were necessary for happiness, but she was motivated now and I knew she could do it, if only she persisted.

• • •

LIKE MANY PEOPLE with traumatic early childhoods, Kestrel carries scars. She steers away from intimacy and is easily enraged by authority figures or anyone who tries to limit her freedom. When she feels pushed, her frosty blue eyes flash fire and she is ready to do battle.

Some nights she attends Pride events, but most nights she stays in her apartment. Before she quit drinking, Kestrel could keep herself entertained with a bottle of red wine and a good movie. But now that she is abstinent, she is jumpy and wound up all the time. She can't sleep more than a few hours a night.

Sex with Becca helps, but Becca wants more from her than sex. Kestrel doesn't like complicated messy relationships. When Becca wants cuddling and affection, Kestrel grows colder. Becca is hurt and they separate for a few days, then Becca calls and suggests a meet up. Kestrel agrees, but only if the relationship stays casual.

Over the years Kestrel has been through this cycle with many partners. This time she is struggling more than usual. Becca is engaging and kind. She tells funny and touching stories about her students, and she works on Pride events with Kestrel.

When Becca goes home after sex, Kestrel finds herself both relieved and disappointed. She is confused about her emotions. Is she feeling this way because she stopped drinking or because Becca is different?

Kestrel's brothers and their families live in Southern California. She sees them occasionally, but she doesn't count on them for anything. Kestrel sees her mother, who lives a couple of hours from her, but she doesn't share information about her emotional or social life. The two of them never talk about their shared traumatic past.

Still, when Evelyn was in her seventies, she often visited Seattle, where Kestrel treated her to ethnic restaurants and musicals. Evelyn enjoyed this immensely and could be effusive in her pleasures. When she drank champagne she was as giggly as a girl; and when she and Kestrel went to the theater for musicals, she would sing on the way home. Evelyn is in her eighties now and too frail to travel, but she and Kestrel talk on the phone once a week. This is as close as Kestrel comes to a commitment.

Kestrel wouldn't describe herself as lonely. She sees herself as a self-sufficient person who likes privacy. She is a stranger to the joys of self-disclosure and trust.

• • •

No MATTER THE reasons why we are lonely, we can always find ways to connect with others. We can commit ourselves to going out at least once a day and to talking with the people we encounter in the stores or along our route. We can chat with the woman who is walking her dog or the mother with young children in the park. We can call a relative or an old friend or do volunteer work. One of our best strategies is to think of someone who is lonely, then give her a call.

We need one person who consistently cares about us. Or as my friend Alberta put it, "I want someone to give a damn about how my day went." For many of us, our significant other is a close woman friend. We are lucky if we have a safety net of friends. But, if we don't, we can build such a community. We can find a place of worship, set up a weekly coffee hour, invite our neighbors over for beans-and-rice night, or join an existing group.

A community of friends becomes an extended family. These communities give us what we could call "rituals of survival," ways to connect with others and hold our lives in place. No matter what age we are, to be fully human we need to feel embedded in community. As my brother Jake says, "We are all just baby mice, huddled together to stay warm."

Social scientists know that it is essential to love and feel loved. A study published in early 2015 by Brigham Young University found that isolation and loneliness are as bad for health as smoking fifteen cigarettes a day or being an alcoholic. Especially in this life stage, none of us can totally avoid loneliness. However, we can view it as a signal to nurture ourselves and to reach out to others.

We can also learn to alchemize loneliness into solitude. We can reframe the time we spend alone as positive time and find more ways to enjoy ourselves. We can listen to music, watch movies, read, or engage in creative pursuits. We can decide to make ourselves a delicious healthy meal every night using new recipes. Or we can take up a new interest such as photography, scrapbooking, or genealogy.

By using our memories, we can visit all of the people in our past. When I feel blue, I remember my grandmothers and aunts, or my best friends from junior high, high school, or college. I recall trips with my closest friends and all the fun times we have shared. I envision vacations and long conversations in good restaurants. I remember the many times I've felt cherished by my adult children and grandchildren. One night when I couldn't sleep I tried to recall every boy I'd ever kissed. That was fun.

Books are great companions. When we read, we can share our day with Anna Karenina, Madame Bovary, or Jane Eyre. We can travel all over the world and live in all times and places. We can dine with Mary and Percy Shelley in Italy or Simone de Beauvoir and Gertrude Stein in Paris.

Book groups celebrate reading. Members enjoy social time, but also the opportunity to discuss serious ideas and multiple points of view. Members help each other find and select the best of readings, and most women in book groups report that they read more because of the inspiration of their groups.

Many a woman has been comforted by her relationship to her cat or dog. Beloved pets take care of us even as they allow us to care for them. Walking our dog gives us a reason to get out of the house and a way to get to know other people we encounter on our walks. Sleeping beside a purring cat is the equivalent of three glasses of wine. Note: I just made that up, but, based on my experience, it seems about right.

We older women are likely to possess many of the skills we need to enjoy alone time. We have built them over the decades. But, with new challenges, we will need to acquire even more skills.

After her husband's death, Marta discovered new ways to connect with her children. Marta and John had opened a small engine repair shop in Cleveland almost fifty years ago when they were first married and starting a family. John died last year. After his funeral, Marta closed the shop for a week and then reopened it. She could repair motors and replace blades as well as John could. She felt less lonely at work than she did at home.

The shop wasn't busy, but when people came in, they were usually old customers with time to visit. When Marta wasn't waiting on customers, she tinkered with machines or read the local paper. She played bluegrass and country music tapes on an old boom box that John had given her one birthday.

Marta had two children, a daughter who lived in Dallas and a son in Dayton. Hannah was thirty, single, and working in payroll for a large department store. Earl was a mechanic with a teenage son named Curtis and a wife who was not fond of Marta. Jodi considered Marta a terrible cook and housekeeper. Marta agreed, but she didn't understand why that was important. Jodi couldn't change a tire or unstop a drain and Marta didn't hold this against her. Marta seldom saw either of her children, and at first, she didn't mind. She didn't miss them much; she missed John.

Hannah called her every Sunday night. She'd ask about Marta, then tell her about her problems at work or with her apartment. Marta looked forward to these calls, which grew a little longer every Sunday. One night, to her own surprise, Marta offered to pay airfare for Hannah to come visit every few months. Hannah said she would and they scheduled the first visit since John's funeral.

Some Saturdays Earl and his son drove over for a visit. They'd play horseshoes or go bowling and then eat out at a steak house. Curtis would graduate from high school next year. He wanted to go to college, but the family didn't have money saved. Marta offered him a place to stay if he attended school in Cleveland. Curtis looked grateful and said he'd think about it.

A few weeks later, Marta called Curtis and asked if he'd like to work in the shop with her after school was out. She said she could use the company and would teach him what she knew about fixing things. She offered to pay him whatever he would have made in his hometown over the summer. Curtis said he'd like to. He was ready to live in a big city. When she hung up, Marta danced a jig.

Some women easily master the art of living alone. Estelle runs a successful medical supply business. She learned her profession from her first employer, and by the time she was thirty she had saved enough money to start her own small business in North Omaha. Now she has five stores in the metropolitan area. She also advises young entrepreneurs in the African American community.

Estelle lives in a condo downtown with her German shepherd dog, Mingus. She works with people all day and is happy to come home to a quiet place and a loving pet. She doesn't see her friends most nights; she prefers solitude. On weekend nights, she sometimes goes out to dinner or to concerts with her gal pals. On Saturdays, she sees her sister, Melva, who lives in the suburbs of Omaha. The two are close, although their old family roles still cause some conflict. Estelle is the big sister who tends to offer advice. Melva can be the bratty younger sister who doesn't care to be told what to do. Still, they text each other constantly and Estelle takes vacations with Melva and her two daughters. She hired one of her nieces to work for her. She wants to teach her the business and some day to turn it over to her.

On Sundays, Estelle visits her sixty-year-old brother, Ike, who lives in a rehabilitation center near downtown Omaha. When he was in his forties, he was in a car accident and broke his neck. Since then, he's lived at Riverview. Estelle brings him audiobooks and hard candies. She also brings Mingus, who is much loved by Ike and the other residents. There is even an outdoor courtyard for pleasant days.

On days when the weather is good Estelle wheels Ike to an outdoor courtyard for a picnic. Some Saturdays Estelle and Ike watch football on TV and other days they play Scrabble. Estelle tells Ike about work problems. He's a good listener and, on the rare occasion when he makes a suggestion, Estelle usually likes it.

Estelle doesn't wish she were married or had children, but sometimes she does wish she had someone to cook her meals and give her kisses. Instead, she walks Mingus, checks her Facebook, or reads blogs and news magazines. She no longer dates—too many issues from income, race, gender, and politics to concerns about sexually transmitted diseases and sexual expectations. At her age, she thinks that most of the available men aren't up to her standards. Besides, she has Ike, Melva, the nieces, and a few good friends.

Depending on our personalities and circumstances, we can all find ways to cope with loneliness. One of my friends spends her days studying up on policy issues that affect her city and state. Then she meets with the appropriate officials to share her information and opinions. She eats lunch every day in the cafeteria at city hall so that she can rub shoulders with lawmakers and be a person of influence. Another bought a small time-share in Santa Fe and invites her friends to come down and explore the area with her.

Twice a year Jean travels with group tours to learn more about history. In between trips, she reads up on the place she'll be visiting. Her most recent trip was to Vietnam. Sometimes she finds a friend to accompany her, but by now she is brave enough to go alone and trust that she'll make friends on the tour.

Even if we have been lifelong extroverts, most of us enjoy solitude as we grow older. One of the secrets of happiness is having a host of activities that we can enjoy when we are alone. The more we can do this, the more likely we are to enjoy our lives as we age. When we use our skills for self-nourishment and to foster deeper connections with the people who remain in our lives, loneliness transforms into solitude. Let's now examine the specific skills we need as we journey on.

PART II

TRAVEL
SKILLS

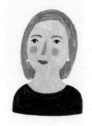

CHAPTER 8

Understanding Ourselves

"A woman is like a tea bag—you can't tell how strong she is
until you put her in hot water." —Eleanor Roosevelt

"Nobody will protect you from your suffering.
You can't cry it away or eat it away or starve it away or walk it
away or punch it away or even therapy it away. It's just there,
and you have to survive it. You have to endure it. You have to
live through it and love it and move on and be better for it and
run as far as you can . . . across the bridge that was built by
your own desire to heal." —Cheryl Strayed

LONG AGO MY seventeen-year-old niece called from a convenience store
in Oklahoma to tell me she was lost. This was years before we had GPS
devices, and my niece didn't even have a map. She knew she was not on
the right road and she asked me how to drive to Lincoln from where she

was. I pulled out a map and asked where she was. Unfortunately, she didn't know.

"Let's start by asking the clerk at the Kwik Stop what town you are in," I told her. "You can't navigate from there to here if you don't know where you are."

That is the situation we older women are always in. Our lives are changing constantly in significant ways and knowing where we are is a much more complicated question than simply knowing our geographical location. It means having a strong sense of ourselves and our own needs in shifting situations. That requires the skill of paying attention to that voice deep inside that wants to take good care of us.

Of course, we can't understand ourselves completely. We are all stymied by ignorance, confusion, and limited points of view. Defenses, such as denial, cognitive dissonance, projection, and compartmentalization, prevent us from understanding everything.

We are also constrained by the ways we are taught to think, feel, and behave and by our culture's definitions of our roles. In fact, one mark of wisdom is the ability to distinguish between who we are educated to be and who we truly are.

We can talk to friends or therapists about our struggles. We can participate in various kinds of groups, such as women's groups, that foster self-awareness. We can journal or meditate. We can read psychology books or, my personal favorite, we can simply walk or sit and think.

The more we understand ourselves, the more skilled we will be at distinguishing between acting on impulse and listening to the nurturing voice deep inside us that says, "This is important to you." The more self-knowledge we have the more likely it is that we will be able to act in accordance with our truest selves.

To grow into our largest best selves, we must be able to claim our own lives. We need to sort out what we truly desire and then go for it.

This kind of empowerment for women is almost always hard-won. Our culture educates us to be responsible, nurturing, and available to others. We must learn on our own to take care of ourselves.

Whenever someone needed my mother, her mother, or my aunts, they would say automatically, "Duty calls" or "Your wish is my command." Of course, duty will always call, but we need not respond automatically the way the women in my mother's family did. Before we leap to engage with whoever wants our services, we can allow ourselves the freedom to think about our decisions.

We can learn to protect our time and space. Time management is not for the faint of heart. Life has a way of getting complicated and messy. Simplicity in life is as difficult to achieve as clarity is in writing. One powerful skill is learning to make position statements. These are statements about what we will and will not do. "I am too busy for houseguests" is not a position statement. "I am not going to host any more company this year" is a position statement. Another might be "I don't take calls after dinnertime" or "I reserve Sundays for family dinners." When we first do this, it feels as if we are breaking a taboo. However, afterward, we experience a rush of newfound freedom.

The power of "no" is hard-won. As women, we learn to say phrases like "Maybe later" or "I'll think about that" or "Yes, that would be okay." In fact, we have no training to simply say no. The first time that I had a request to do something I didn't want to do and the word "no" popped out of my mouth, I thought lightning would strike me dead. It felt so weird to actually tell the truth in a direct way without modifiers. I still mostly soften and modify my denials, but whenever I use the word "no," I feel a burst of power and joy.

The power of "yes" consists of affirming our own needs. This is a new skill for many women even at sixty-five. First, we need to know our own needs, and then be assertive enough to say what they are, even when this may inconvenience others. It is challenging to say, "I want this, and I am going to make it happen." However, if we can learn to do this, we will be able to make intentional choices about our time.

We can grant ourselves the power to walk out of any room we don't want to be in. When I look back over my life, I can recall multiple times when I felt I was being badly treated. A supervisor was yelling at me, a friend was berating me unjustly, or I was being "coached" in a way that made me deeply embarrassed and ashamed. In every one of those cases I wish I'd had the strength to simply walk out of the room. Since I discovered this new power, I do not stay in any situation in which I feel neglected, discounted, or disrespected. I infrequently walk out, but knowing I have that option makes me feel safer.

• • •

EVEN THOUGH REDHEADS are stereotyped as hot-tempered, Emma has a long history of accommodating her family, especially her daughter, Alice. Raised in a traditional family in rural Colorado, Emma learned to be a "good girl" and to hold herself responsible for the emotions of everyone around her. This upbringing has caused her lots of trouble. When she strives to make everyone happy, she loses herself. After a day of serving others, Emma sometimes feels bitter that she isn't more appreciated and valued.

Her down-to-earth husband, Chris, was raised on a farm in Wyoming. Emma takes good care of him and in return he is the rock that tethers her rather directionless kite to the earth. Mostly this is a good thing for her, but sometimes Chris's practicality and consistency irritate her. Chris gets frustrated by what he calls Emma's scatterbrained nature. When their bank account is low and Emma gives money to Alice, he blows up.

She and Alice tense up around each other. In some ways they are too much alike and in other ways they are polar opposites. Alice is a big spender and quite self-absorbed. Emma admires her spunk and ability to take care of herself, but she also sees Alice as ungrateful and thoughtless. She has no idea how to negotiate with Alice or how to ask for her respect.

Emma's greatest struggle is to listen to her own voice and to act on what it tells her she truly needs and wants. She was socialized to believe that good women were happy only when others were happy and to monitor the room and take emotional responsibility for all of the feelings in it. No one ever taught her to take care of herself.

In addition to her lack of a strong centerboard, Emma has all the sorrows of most women in our life stage. Her friends are beginning to fall ill or move away to the warmth of Arizona. Both of her parents are gone now, and she misses her mother terribly. She despairs about politics and worries about the future of the planet. She wants a healthy peaceful place for her grandchildren and for everyone else's children too. She grinds her teeth at night.

Every morning when Emma says her prayers, she aspires to be grateful and present. However, like most of us, she finds that much harder than she wishes it were. There are so many things that can take her off course and leave her jangled and forgetful.

Her optimistic predictions and endlessly high expectations are often dashed by reality. More than once, she has looked forward to a family holiday only to dissolve in tears when the last family member said goodbye. Or, she has anticipated an outing with Alice only to be disappointed when she cancels or shows up with an impatient or even hostile attitude.

One night, after writing Alice a rent check and fixing her family dinner, Emma broke down while she washed dishes. Alice hadn't even thanked her. Not only that, Alice had hugged Chris goodbye while pointedly ignoring Emma.

Chris stopped drying the dishes and patted Emma awkwardly and said gently, "I hope that rent check doesn't bounce."

Emma sobbed for an hour. She was filled with self-pity, guilt, and bitterness. She knew that she couldn't please everyone and realized in her heart what a futile desire that was.

Emma found a therapist her age who listened carefully as Emma talked about her struggles with her family. Laurel asked questions, then observed, "I notice your breathing is shallow. Let me help you with that."

Laurel taught her some deep breathing and centering exercises. She also recommended that Emma find a yoga class and schedule a monthly massage. Laurel encouraged Emma to focus on her body, breathing, and heart.

Until her first massage, Emma had no idea how tense she was. Afterward, she was sore all over, but she almost skipped to her car. Over time, with a yoga class and massage, Emma grew more familiar with her own body.

Laurel taught her mindfulness skills. They began and ended sessions with meditation and sometimes paused during a session for a minute meditation. Emma learned to look inside herself and explore her inner landscape. She realized how guilt-ridden and opinionated she was. Laurel helped her examine all of this without judgment. Over time Emma became more able to hear her own true voice.

By the time she stopped therapy, Emma could pay attention to that inner balk that she sometimes felt when people asked her for one more favor. Slowly she is learning that when she feels tired and reluctant to do something, that is time for her to say no. Often she says, "Let me think about that and get back to you." That gives her even more space to consider her own needs.

Emma has weeks when she is more centered, focused, and assertive, and then she will fail miserably for a while. She can be so other-focused that she can't remember to breathe deeply or pause before responding to requests. Still, she has made progress on knowing her own boundaries and paying attention to her own body, heart, and mind.

• • •

SELF-KNOWLEDGE AND SELF-PROTECTIVE skills become even more important as we age. If we are not frozen in denial, we are likely to feel anguish on a regular basis. Emotions offer information that we want to receive gratefully and attend carefully.

Pain is a natural and healthy reaction to distress, necessary for survival. When we cut our finger, it bleeds. That is what is supposed to happen. When we unblock dammed-up emotions, we allow a fresh stream of vitality to flow through us. Whether we are grieving the loss of a beloved or are upset about a daily event, we want to experience our emotions in our hearts, minds, and bodies. Darkness experienced honestly and openly becomes less overwhelming. None of us do this perfectly or all the time. What counts is the effort we make to know ourselves.

I met Meredith on a long flight down the East Coast. She was from Georgia and spoke with a Southern accent. She was an attractive woman who at sixty-six still had smooth skin dotted with freckles. When I told her I was a psychologist and writer, she wanted to talk about her divorce.

I asked her permission to interview her and pulled out a pen and paper. The first opportunity she had, she ordered a Scotch on the rocks. Perhaps because of the drink and her passion for her topic, she talked loudly in an animated way. I was concerned that other passengers could hear her story, but she didn't seem to mind.

Meredith had been divorced for fifteen years, but she talked about it as if it had happened yesterday. She had been a naïve young woman studying nursing when she met Doug at a party. He was a calm engineering major. She told me, "Doug liked my social ease and chattiness.

I liked his solidity." Then she snorted and said, "It turned out to be rigidity and stubbornness."

After Meredith ordered her second drink, she explained to me that Doug was not an expressive person. She hoped she could teach him to communicate his feelings. She shook her head and said, "Don't we all think we're going to change them?"

They married in 1975. Meredith had some reservations before the wedding, but she ignored them. She told me, "The only things we had in common were the St. Louis Cardinals and the Rolling Stones."

From the beginning the marriage was tense. "I carry my emotions one eighth of an inch below the surface of my skin," she explained. "Doug couldn't stand what he called my 'extroverting all over him.' I couldn't discover his love language, and I don't think he even looked for mine."

Doug insisted that both of them work and save. After their daughters were born, he encouraged Meredith to return to work as soon as she could. He traveled for an oil company and, when he was home, he was unwilling to spend money on movies or family vacations.

One year Doug didn't make it home for Meredith's birthday. A few weeks later, he confessed that he was having an affair. Meredith fell apart and cried for three days. She recorded her sobs and sent them to Doug in an email. He didn't respond.

Meredith was filled with regrets and rage and couldn't stop feeling like a fool. Finally, she filed for divorce. "It was a long and bitter process, and the bitterness isn't over," she hissed.

Doug married the woman from Texas. Meredith remained in Atlanta, working as a nurse and caring for her daughters. Doug made almost no effort to see them and they didn't miss him much.

After her youngest daughter left for college, Meredith bought some sexy clothes and had what she called a "tramp stamp" tattooed on her lower back. She hadn't dated in decades, but plunged into online dating. She fell for one man, slept with him, and was hurt by his rejection two weeks later. Other men were so lonely that they proposed after one or two dates. One man turned out to be a stalker and she had to call the police for a restraining order. For now, she has quit dating altogether.

When the pilot announced that we were twenty minutes from the airport, I thanked her for talking to me so honestly. I gently suggested that perhaps a therapist could be of use to her. I said, "I think you are giving your ex-husband too much power over your present life."

Meredith shook her head as if she were coming out of a trance. She rearranged her face to look as it had when I sat down beside her. It was the face of the placid, confident woman. But I knew better.

How many of us learn to arrange our faces this way? How many of us look different from the way we are feeling inside? How many of us are carrying heavy burdens of anger and regret?

Meredith was seeking to understand herself by having an alcohol-fueled conversation with a stranger. I respect that she was trying. All our efforts are commendable. We cannot make choices, face challenges, or build good days without some sense for what we are experiencing. Only then can we discover where we are going and how to move toward our destination.

One of our greatest challenges may be learning to deal with all the anger that we've carried for decades. We've lived in a deeply patriarchal culture all of our lives and we've been encouraged to bury our anger and smile our way through life. When we are harassed by men, or find ourselves placating a man who is criticizing us, we store our anger in our bodies. However, for women of our generation, anger is an especially difficult emotion to experience. It's so "unladylike."

Often our anger turns inward toward depression or toward self-destructive behaviors that leave us enveloped in clouds of shame. Anger, held onto across time, is resentment, and resentment is like swallowing poison and waiting for the other person to die. Or as Jean Améry wrote, resentment "nails every one of us onto the cross of [our own] ruined past."

Many of us find anger to be a deeply dysphoric experience and do our best to move on. Although it can seem counterintuitive, the healthiest way to do this is to allow ourselves to fully experience our anger. Anger is about protecting something vulnerable inside or outside ourselves. Instead of saying, "I am angry," it can be helpful to say, "Anger is happening." This can allow us to be curious about our anger rather than losing ourselves in it.

Experiencing anger is one thing. Knowing how to express it is another. Often, we can find ourselves alternating between rage and stony silence, neither of which is functional. We each must learn, through trial and error, how to voice our anger. The answer to a question about how to express our anger is, "It depends." It depends who we are with, what the situation is, how out-of-control we feel, and what is likely to be the result of our expression of anger. A good question to ask ourselves is, "Are there ways to voice my anger that will benefit me or anyone else?"

Often, what works best is to wait until we have dealt with our anger internally and pondered how best to handle it. But sometimes, it just feels so right to say, "That makes me mad."

It often helps to have physical ways to release anger. Otherwise all of that arousal and energy can stay in the body and keep us agitated. There are many ways to do this. We can pound a pillow, throw ice cubes in our shower, throw stones at a tree, or find something to kick until we are exhausted. When we physically discharge our anger, we experience a cleansing, a catharsis. We calm down and are able to think rationally about the appropriate response to whoever angered us.

Many women our age feel less anger. We have learned how to work with all our negative emotions and deal with relationships more skillfully. We are more accepting of ourselves and other people, and we're better at navigating life's constant challenges. We can keep our boats even-keeled. However, if we have not learned to cope with intense emotions, now is the time to learn, and quickly. As the Buddhists know, life is suffering. We cannot avoid that, but we can strengthen ourselves for the days ahead.

With self-awareness, our own natural vitality, and our many life skills, we can maintain our stubborn zest for life regardless of circumstance. We will feel gratitude and joy even as we accept life as it is. When we learn to do this, we can call ourselves "seasoned" or "vintage." We've grown into the finest of wines.

We will no longer feel the responsibility to fix everything. We won't have as many opinions on how other people should live their lives. Instead we'll expand our moral imaginations to include more points of view.

We'll be less constrained by cultural rules and roles. We will discover talents we did not know we had and find in ourselves untapped reserves of courage and joy. We'll discover ourselves to be bigger people than we had imagined possible.

CHAPTER 9

Making Intentional Choices

"One's philosophy is not best expressed in words; it is expressed in the choices one makes . . . And the choices we make are ultimately our own responsibility." —Eleanor Roosevelt

"There is nothing inevitable. The actions of the past operate in every instant and so, at every instant, does freedom." —Nan Shin

MARLENE GREW UP in a poor family with a father who spent a lot of time at a bar and managed to be so drunk that he was kicked out of his children's weddings. Her mother was a strong woman who supported her deadbeat husband and seven children by working at the school cafeteria. This mom had a sunny disposition and wouldn't tolerate complaints.

When the children were whining or discouraged, she would say, "Buck up, chipmunks."

Marlene is a large woman who wears colorful skirts, lacy blouses, and dangly earrings. She claims she has never lost a cussing contest with anyone. She gives co-workers pet names and she can make almost anyone laugh. Marlene is bright and energetic, like her mother, and she too has led a life of poverty. Because of her epilepsy, she has never been able to drive or work in places where her seizures could create problems. She wanted to work with children or in a hospital as a caregiver but, as she said, "Those jobs were not open to me."

Marlene married and left home early. She doesn't remember a time when she was not working. Now she has a job at a food distribution center and lives in subsidized housing. When she finishes her day, she can pick up groceries for herself and her boyfriend. She has two grown children, a son who is in the military and a daughter who lives in another state.

Marlene divorced their father long ago and swore off men until five years ago when she met Danny. She calls him "my honey" and they spend a great deal of time together. Their favorite television show is *Criminal Minds*. They treat themselves to a fried chicken dinner at a fast-food place every Friday night and they play cards, bingo, and dominoes at her housing complex. Marlene told me that by the time she and Danny met, they both knew what was important. They didn't waste time on bickering or complaining. They made the best of life.

"I decided early that things were going to be tough and I'd better figure out ways to enjoy myself," Marlene said. This intention has shaped her life. Her lifelong poverty and her epilepsy could have made her miserable, but Marlene refused to let that happen. She told me, "I always choose love and joy."

Attitude trumps circumstance. Every woman determines her own history, but not necessarily under conditions that she chooses. We all keep appointments we did not make. Still, we have the freedom to choose how we respond to inner or outer events. Luck is neither a necessary nor a sufficient condition for happiness. Attitude is both.

Happiness is a choice and a set of skills. We all live within the confines of the world as it is but we have the freedom to frame that world in ways that allow us to be positive and grateful. Once we have made the existential choice to be happy, we can develop a repertoire of skills to achieve our goals. It is never too late to become a happier person. Hopelessness and happiness are both self-fulfilling prophecies. We become who we believe we can be.

Recent research by psychologist Sonja Lyubomirsky finds that 50 percent of our happiness may be related to our genetics. The rest is determined by a combination of circumstances, attitude, and actions. According to Lyubomirsky, we can most influence our own happiness by reframing our situations in positive ways, being thankful, and giving to others. We don't have total control, but we have choices. In fact, research in epigenetics reveals that the ways we think about aging can actually impact our DNA as well as many other aspects of our later years.

Some women can be disabled by a hangnail, while others could be hit by a truck and keep smiling. The difference involves attitude and coping capacities. We can learn to define ourselves by our grit and we can learn the skills to make this happen.

We can choose the way we talk to ourselves. We can face reality and acknowledge and explore our own pain, but also tell ourselves, "Things will work out," "I can do it," or "Rome wasn't built in a day." We can count our blessings, find the silver lining, and look on the bright side. By our age, many of us know how to do these things, at least sometimes.

Recently I heard a good message for calming down. My daughter Sara's family and a friend of hers from out of town were over for dinner when Sara's dog ran away. She, her husband, and my husband all went looking for Bix. My grandson Coltrane, the visiting friend, and I waited outside, hoping Bix would return. After a few minutes, Coltrane said in a rather panicky voice, "What if Bix is dead?" I replied, "Bix is okay and he will return soon. The worst thing that could happen is he won't return before we have dinner. That could make everyone stressed during our meal." Sara's friend said simply, "It's not time to worry yet." We all calmed down, and sure enough, Bix ran into our yard in the next five minutes. Since then, on multiple occasions, I have used that phrase, "It's not time to worry yet."

There are many ways to keep things in perspective. We can volunteer at a homeless shelter or a hospice unit. Or we can employ such useful sentences as "It could be worse" or "Tomorrow is another day" or "Everyone makes mistakes."

Natalie has her perspective skills down cold. She is fighting the autoimmune disease lupus, which leads to a low blood cell count with its many accompanying problems. She has had blood transfusions, cellulitis, and injuries from falls and even brushing her teeth. Yet, she told me, "I never give lupus top billing in my life."

Her illness keeps her from coming to many get-togethers, but, when she does return, Natalie labels every event she can a party. She holds scrapbooking, casserole-baking, and clean-up-the-garage parties. She puts on music, starts dancing and, voilà, we are at a party. If I ask Natalie, "Do we have time for a walk, or a cup of coffee, or some picture sharing from our iPhones?" Her answer will always be, "Are you kidding? I always have time for that."

• • •

Dressed in a crisp black business suit, her auburn hair pulled back into a braid, Willow accompanied Saul to a checkup. The doctor reviewed Saul's latest tests and examined him carefully. Then he patted Saul's shoulder and told them that Saul's Parkinson's disease was progressing aggressively. He predicted that Saul would soon be in a wheelchair and have more trouble speaking and swallowing.

That night Willow was so saddened by the doctor's news that she could hardly sleep. She imagined the suffering in Saul's future and fretted about her own ability to cope. But the next morning, she woke up ready to organize. She called her office and said she would not be in all week. Then she made a list of everything in the apartment that needed to change so that Saul could move around without hurting himself.

She hired carpenters and plumbers to install a new shower so that Saul could maneuver more safely. She prepared a grocery list of all the foods that would be easy for Saul to manage. She invited their six closest friends to dinner that Saturday night. She told Saul, "Better to tell them all together and be done with it."

Over the next few weeks, Willow reconsidered her priorities. She had planned to cut back her hours, but keep working. Then, one morning Saul could not get out of bed by himself. She helped him up and to the bathroom, then made coffee for the two of them. While she did this, she decided it was time to quit her job. As she poured the coffee, she wiped tears from her cheeks. It had been such a privilege to be of service to people in need.

Willow called her office and said she would be in for two more days to finish up and say goodbye. Her assistant was less surprised by the news than Willow had been. She said, "We will miss you, but you are making the right decision. The last time I saw Saul, I knew it was time."

When she told Saul the news, he shook his head no, then began to cry. She hugged him and said, "From now on, I want to be with you."

As the months passed, Willow wondered how the agency was doing. Once a week she had lunch with the new director and talked about the many issues that come up with a nonprofit. She stopped by occasionally to see her old staff and clients. Sometimes she bought street food for Ruby, Myron, and herself. She missed the job, but she didn't regret her decision.

Willow had new tasks now, as Saul's caretaker, nurse, and scheduler. She cut his food for him and helped him on and off the toilet. She managed his medications and helped him bathe and get dressed. She selected films for them to watch at home and invited friends to come visit on a weekly rotation.

The most stressful aspect of Saul's illness for Willow was decision-making. She was an interventionist who wanted to implement everything that might help Saul. He tended to resist treatment or any activities that required energy. Eventually, though, Saul established that *he* would be the decider about his own health.

At first, Willow could hardly stand to keep silent. She was tense around doctors' appointments because they carried potential for conflict. But over time, she reframed her role from being his nurse to being his nurturer. She decided that the most important thing for her was to keep their relationship strong and loving. She told Saul, "Whatever you choose to do or not do about your health, I will be there for you."

When Willow thought about the future, she was frightened, but most of the time she lived in a day-to-day, problem-solving mode. She tried to make every day a good one. She didn't want to be at war with reality. Rather, she wanted to face it, befriend it, and learn from it.

Willow's choices changed her. She entered the most spiritually intense time of her life. She grew less task-oriented and more inclined to laugh. She discovered that she liked herself and other people more than ever before. Even as she grieved at Saul's diminished health, she felt awake and grateful. Listening to Rachmaninoff or watching the sunset over the park could be blissful. For the first time in her life, Willow felt fully alive.

• • •

FREEDOM IS THE ability to make conscious choices in accord with our deepest values. It is the opposite of reactivity, which we could define as acting on every whim, impulse, and emotion that we experience. Reactivity leads us to self-destructive choices. Freedom requires self-awareness and the skill of choosing where to place our attention and how to frame the circumstances we find ourselves in.

We all feel hopeless at times. Events have the power to knock us to our knees. Even with self-awareness, it's too much to expect that our response to everything be transcendent. We all grow weary of trying. Or, as one of my friends put it, "I am so damn tired of these fucking growth experiences."

However, we can move toward acceptance and resilience. And our tragedies can teach us to trust and connect us to others.

This happened to Kestrel early in May when her mother called her at work. In a trembling voice, Evelyn said, "I have stage III lung cancer. Please come home. I want you to be with me at the doctor's office tomorrow."

Fifteen minutes later, Kestrel was driving from downtown Seattle toward her hometown, her frosty blue eyes laser focused on the road. At the appointment, Kestrel took notes while she and her mother listened to the doctor's report. He recommended surgery followed by radiation therapy. When he finished, he looked Evelyn in the eyes and said softly, "I am sorry."

Kestrel and Evelyn held hands for a few minutes without speaking. The doctor sat quietly too. Finally, Kestrel said, "We need to talk before we make decisions."

When they arrived home, Kestrel made Evelyn peppermint tea and they sat in the garden watching long shadows creep across the lawn. After dinner, Evelyn went to bed early and Kestrel allowed herself the luxury of a bike ride on her old Schwinn. She peddled around town looking at her childhood landscape. Everything seemed smaller and dingier.

When she rode past the school where she and her brothers had been teased, Kestrel felt a wave of anger. When she looked at the grocery store where her family always owed money, she felt shame. So many of her memories of this town were unhappy ones. She thought, "No wonder I've been angry all my life."

However, as she biked on, she had another thought: "But who exactly has my anger been punishing?"

The next morning, Kestrel did medical research on the Internet. Over a lunch of chili and cinnamon rolls, Kestrel reminded her mother that she had choices and that Evelyn, not the doctor, was in charge of her care. Evelyn warned Kestrel to take it easy on her doctor. She said, "I need to believe he can help me."

Kestrel looked at her frightened mother and said, "Okay, Mom. I trust him, but you still call the shots."

Evelyn decided to schedule the surgery her doctor recommended. While she called the nurse to do this, Kestrel wrapped her arms around her mother. She clung to her through the entire call. Kestrel wasn't sure who was comforting whom.

The next day Kestrel took a leave of absence from her technology company and called Becca to explain that she would be away all summer. Becca was so empathic and kind that Kestrel realized she would miss her. That thought made her nervous. She didn't like being vulnerable to others.

In the days before her mother's surgery, Kestrel bought groceries, did laundry, and planted some day lilies in her mother's garden. One morning she and her mom looked at old family picture albums, but those did not make them happy. So instead they did crosswords and listened to Evelyn's records from the 1950s, mostly musicals and big bands. At night, Kestrel contended with her desire to raid her mother's small liquor cabinet. She didn't know how to handle so much pain.

The evening after Evelyn's surgery, when Kestrel was home alone, she was tempted to drink her mother's vodka. Instead, she called Becca, who encouraged her to talk about her emotions. At first, Becca's suggestion made Kestrel irritated, but soon she found herself opening up to Becca. She said she was angry that God would put someone so sweet and good through cancer treatments. She hated that much of her mother's life had been miserable. Kestrel's intensity didn't scare Becca. She simply listened. When Kestrel hung up, she felt anxious about her self-disclosure, but also relieved that she had actually told someone about her pain. She was surprised at how easy it had been to talk.

Evelyn returned home from surgery tired and sore. She had pain pills, but only took one of them before she turned to ibuprofen. She spent several days dozing in sunbeams or doing crossword puzzles in the garden. Kestrel fielded calls from her brothers, the pharmacist, and the doctor's office. She helped her mother bathe and move from room to room.

She called Becca every night for support. Sometimes they talked about her mother's cancer, but other times Becca would tell her the news from their activist group and about her day at work. Kestrel thought Becca had a lovely ability to make an ordinary day seem fun and exciting.

After much discussion, Evelyn had her first radiation treatment. It left her with diarrhea, vomiting, and weakness. When she felt better, Evelyn decided not to return for a second treatment. She wasn't afraid of dying, and she didn't want to suffer any more.

One afternoon, when Kestrel brought her a bouquet from the garden, Evelyn told her that she had enjoyed a wonderful summer. "My favorite times have always been with you. This summer of cancer was no exception."

Kestrel swallowed hard, her frosty blue eyes soft and kind. She said, "I love you, Mom."

• • •

WE CAN BE intentional in a hundred different ways. We can commit to a trusting relation or a volunteer project. We can decide whom we spend time with, when we will retire, where we will live, and how we will spend our valuable resources. Time is the most valuable resource of all. Ultimately, all our most important decisions are about time. What will we do with our mornings, afternoons, evenings, days, and weeks?

When we are in our twenties, thirties, and forties, children and/or work can keep us rushed and scheduled. During these earlier decades, we are more likely to make reactive choices. We have a work deadline, the baby needs to go to the doctor, or the third-grader needs help with his spelling test. Mothers of school-age children tend to pack lunches, supervise teeth brushing, and attend parent-teacher conferences and soccer practices. We buy groceries, wash clothes, cook meals, and tell bedtime stories. Time spends us and leaves us spent.

As we age, more of us have the opportunity for reflective decision-making around time. We can learn to kayak, take exercise or cooking classes, or volunteer to teach English to refugees. We can regularly examine our current routines and habits and decide whether they are enjoyable or just, well, habitual. We can set priorities and separate the essential from the nonessential. We can ask, "Am I spending my time in accordance with my values?" or "When I look back on my life at the end, will I feel good about how I parceled out my small measure of time?"

Each of us has the freedom to decide what is essential. A recent Nielsen survey found that retired people spend an average of fifty hours a week watching television. The women who do this are missing chances to be engaged with others and develop their many gifts.

We can be intentional in our use of money or other kinds of wealth. My definition of wealth has varied across the years from the number of nights a year I sleep outside to the number of days a month I see my grandchildren. Another definition that I favor is the number of people I am in loving relationships with. We are educated by the culture to believe that security comes from money, but really, in this life stage, what saves most of us is love. We can all write our own definitions of wealth. When we do this, it clarifies what it is we are trying to accumulate.

Of course, some women consider wealth to be the money in their bank accounts. And, certainly, financial security is conducive to a comfortable, secure life. However, women with money can still feel poor because they are unable to define the word "enough," and thus remain haunted by scarcity.

It's important to distinguish between wants and needs. When our needs are met, we have enough. Depending on our finances, we may have choices about what to want. In America, because of our expensive and unpredictable health care system, we are all uncertain that we will have enough for every contingency, but at some point, feeling financially secure means being able to say, "I am not going to worry about this anymore."

One aspect of feeling wealthy is enjoying what one has. Today happens to be a snowy day, and I look out the window every few minutes to just savor the soft white flakes. I sleep under quilts from my grandmother and aunts. I don't store them in a closet. These quilts help me fall asleep; I feel wrapped in grandmothers.

Samantha and her husband, Tony, ran a small art supply store. She is perhaps the most intentional woman I know. On a sunny morning, we talked about her life choices. Samantha and Tony have experienced more than their share of challenges. Tony's father and all of his brothers died young from heart problems. When he was in his mid-sixties, Tony suffered a heart attack while shoveling snow on his driveway.

While he was still in the hospital, he and Samantha decided to sell the shop and retire early. Money would be tight, but time was tighter. A few months later, they were taking pottery classes together at the senior center.

Samantha had experienced cancer twice. The first time, she was thirty-nine years old and the children were in grade school. "Lymphoma was a terrifying thing," she told me. "I asked myself, 'What did I do wrong? Why did this happen to me?' Then I did some bargaining: 'Let me live until they're eighteen.'

"I focused on the treatment and I never broke down emotionally. I didn't cry for six months. Then, when I got the call that my last scan was clear, I fell to pieces. I called Tony at work and I was sobbing so hard I couldn't talk. He thought it was bad news." She laughed and said, "Good news was what made me cry."

When Samantha was diagnosed four years ago with breast cancer, she felt less frightened than she had been after her earlier diagnosis. Her children were grown and she'd whupped cancer before. One day she was driving past the Pink Sisters Chapel. This is a place of utter silence where Sister Servants of the Holy Spirit of Perpetual Adoration, dressed in pink habits, pray nonstop for people from all over the world. Samantha wasn't a Catholic, but something compelled her to go in. She walked into the chapel, where three people were kneeling and a woman lay on the floor flat on her face with her arms out in the sign of the cross.

Samantha sat down and looked at what she believed was a statue of a woman praying. Finally, she realized it was a nun. In the hour Samantha was there, this nun never moved. Samantha said, "The air even seemed to be different there. I became totally calm."

That incident took away any fear she had of this second cancer. Her treatment went well and within months Samantha was once again cancer-free. Even though both cancers could reoccur, Samantha didn't dwell on that: "Because that's like inviting it in. I just proceed as if it's not going to be part of my life."

Samantha has never let illness define her. She says, "We've had some rough stretches but they are background. My new grandson is foreground.

"We've enjoyed every stage of our lives," she continued. "We enjoyed our kids' growing up. When they were babies, we loved them. When they were toddlers, we loved them. We savored every stage, but we were happy to move on to the next. We enjoyed the freedom of being empty nesters. We like it when the kids come home. We like it when they leave."

Samantha and Tony have planned for aging. They don't want to be a burden to their children, who have lives elsewhere. They will remain in their hometown where they have a tremendous support system. Samantha said, "We'd like to just be carried out of our home feet first."

Samantha and Tony are already thinning their load. When their parents died, they inherited more stuff than they wanted or could find room for. They learned that gifts could be unwelcome, no matter how well-meaning. Samantha knows that their children don't want their old stuff either. So, they are asking their adult children to choose what they want. They'll document that and start shedding nonessentials.

"I have no fears of growing older," Samantha told me. "I think I can adjust as it comes along."

Samantha's considered choices have given her a good life in spite of multiple health challenges. She has made the best of it. We can all choose lives that allow us to grow, to love, and to flourish. We can act in ways that we will remember with pride and happiness on our deathbeds. And, almost every morning we can build a good day for ourselves.

CHAPTER 10

Building a Good Day

"One of the secrets of a happy life is continuous small treats."
—Iris Murdoch

"Habit has a kind of poetry." —Simone de Beauvoir

WHEN I WAS a six-year-old living in Beaver City, Nebraska, I read an advertisement for a dog in a teacup. It promised that if I sent a dollar to a post-office box in New York City, a tiny puppy would arrive within ten days. I begged my mother for the required dollar. She warned me that the ad was a hoax, and I would lose my dollar, but I insisted. I wanted that puppy!

After I mailed my envelope, I named the puppy Caramel. Every afternoon I waited on my front porch for the mail carrier. When he showed up without a box, I was deeply disappointed. After ten days my mother suggested I give up hope, but I didn't. I anticipated that puppy for months. In fact, I think a part of me is still waiting.

I no longer send money for puppies in the mail. Most of the time I can manage my expectations. I don't give my adult children unsolicited advice and expect them to appreciate it. I don't expect anyone, including myself, to be good-natured all the time. I love who I love, not only in spite of their flaws, but also because these flaws are an essential part of who they are. And I'm aware that the people who love me are equally merciful.

I don't look at my horoscope; I know what I need to do to be happy.

Building a good day is about making good choices involving our emotions, thinking, and behavior. We can craft days with meaningful activities, satisfying routines, and time with friends and family, and acquire coping strategies that allow us to deal with stress. We can cultivate our sense of humor and, as we sense the fierce urgency of time, we can learn to see our own life in proportion to the whole of life in order to feel grateful simply to be alive.

To be happy we need to learn how to structure a day that is rich in meaning and joy-producing activities. How we spend our time defines who we are. There is no magical future. Today is our future. Our lives are events that unfurl in real time, minute by minute. Right up there with the need for oxygen, food, and sleep is the need to have a reason to get out of bed every morning. We want to be able to think of events we are looking forward to and activities that will give the day a sense of purpose. If we can envision these things, we can find the energy to face even a difficult day.

Many of us wake up grumpy with negative first thoughts. We are likely to think about our worries or our to-do lists for the day. We may have aches and pains. If the weather is gray and cold or we are anticipating unpleasant events, we can be gloomy. However, it's possible to do a mental reset by asking ourselves what we are looking forward to and what we are grateful for.

In life, as in writing, it is as important to know what to delete as it is to know what to add. We don't want our lives to be one long to-do list filled with shoulds and musts. If we are overscheduled and rushing, everything becomes one more chore. When the sunset blazes copper and gold, we don't want to be checking Facebook. When our grandchild asks for a story, we don't want to be preoccupied with paying bills.

We don't want to trudge through our lives doing one dreary chore after another. We want small treats in every day. When times get tough, we want to buy ourselves roses or chocolate bars, make sure we play with our pet, or see our best friend for coffee. These breaks give us time to reconstitute. We can teach ourselves to simply sit down for fifteen minutes and rest or read.

We need space around space. We don't want too many appointments in one day. We want to move in ways that allow us to be relaxed and content. We can allow ourselves puttering time and hang-out time. We can mark out appointment-free days in our schedules and give ourselves days with no cell phones, social media, or news of the world.

As we age, our goals can be greater than our energy levels. Many of us find ourselves with high needs for stimulation and engagement, but limited stamina. Our energy is a valuable resource that must be wisely allocated. Pacing is key. Otherwise, we can collapse with exhaustion and find ourselves in the doldrums for a few days.

There are many polarities in our lives that call for balance and perspective. We try to balance our needs for solitude and companionship, work and relaxation. We want to be health-focused but not health-obsessed. We want to be both spontaneous and disciplined. These sound like rather abstract issues, but this kind of balancing work comes up every day. Do we spend some time catching up on our chores, or do we go with a friend to a concert? Should we read books we loved but haven't read in decades, or do we read new ones? Should we visit our favorite places from the past, or do we travel to new places? Should we work more hours to build up our retirement account, or cut back to spend time with our grandchildren?

To be calm and happy we need multiple reliable ways to cope with stress. We will either develop good habits for dealing with stress or we will adopt self-destructive habits, such as drinking, drugs, or compulsive shopping or television-watching.

Laura, who cares for an ill sister, sings in her church choir. The rehearsals and the Sunday services take her to a joyful and connected place. Reina works in her garden. If she has a difficult interaction with her husband or adult children, she goes outside and pulls a few weeds or waters her roses. Cara picks up a sketchbook and draws whatever sparks her imagination.

• • •

WITH HER GRIEF about her drug-addicted daughter, her pain from arthritis, and her duties as a custodial grandparent, Sylvia found herself having many more bad days than good ones. After a week of sleepless nights, Sylvia made an appointment at the pain clinic that Dr. Peterson recommended.

She approached the appointment with skepticism but when she arrived, she liked the setting. A waterfall gurgled in the waiting room and the air wasn't sullied by television noise. A young physical therapist called her name and Sylvia followed her into a room full of windows and flowering plants.

Megan listened for an hour as Sylvia talked about her pain and her life situation. She asked good questions and accepted all of Sylvia's answers without judgment. Sylvia wasn't sure anyone could help her, but she didn't see how Megan could hurt her much. Megan suggested that Sylvia select a trusted person and, a few minutes a day, talk with them about her pain. To her own surprise, Sylvia immediately said, "I will talk to Lewis. He won't mind listening."

Megan also recommended she rate her pain on a one-to-ten scale and journal about it. Sylvia had never written in a journal or used the pain scale, but these suggestions weren't expensive or invasive. With her lively grandchildren, Sylvia wasn't sure she could find time for a journal, but rating her pain cost her no time at all. As she said goodbye, Sylvia made another appointment.

At the next session Sylvia told Megan that she'd followed through on the suggestions and found them helpful. Rating her pain helped her put it in perspective. The five-minute conversations with Lewis had somehow reconnected them. He occasionally patted her arm now and once even swatted her playfully on the butt. When she said that, they both laughed.

Megan showed Sylvia a few simple back exercises and recommended a homeopathic tea. When Sylvia told her that she had always liked to swim, the therapist offered to arrange for her to swim in the heated pool at a nearby rehabilitation hospital. She was reasonably sure Sylvia's insurance would pay for this. Sylvia decided her schedule was not too crowded for swimming.

A week later she drove to the rehab center and dove into its heated, sparkling pool. That night, she slept for eight hours and made Lewis and the kids pancakes for breakfast. Now, twice a week she leaves Lewis with the children and soothes her mind and body in that lovely water.

For the first time in her life, Sylvia wrote about her own needs and personal priorities. Then she outlined a personal schedule for the week ahead. Of course, she still had Lewis's and the children's schedules in her appointment book but, with red ink, she filled in swimming, back exercises, journaling time, and an hour to go to the women's group at her church.

When she started keeping those red-ink appointments, she began to feel cheerful. Her early pain ratings had been mostly sixes and sevens but now they were twos and threes. She was sleeping better and enjoying her talks with Lewis. Sometimes, after she talked to him, he suggested they play a few hands of gin rummy, and they had some laughs.

Sylvia attended the women's group while the children were in Sunday school. She found herself joking around there just like the Sylvia from long ago. Talking and listening to other women once a week provided her great comfort. She heard how the other women coped with their trials. Some had difficult partners. Two were struggling with cancer. Another suffered recurring spinal fractures from osteoporosis. Sylvia had learned that there was no way to win a suffering contest. Who knew who suffered the most? When she compared her life to her friends' lives, she chose her own.

• • •

JUST AS SYLVIA rated her pain, so can we rate our own stress on a ten-point scale. When we first start doing this, we may rate all of our stressors as elevens, but over time, we learn that real tens are rare occurrences. Most stresses, such as ruining a meal, forgetting an appointment, or losing a library book are only ones and twos. Just being able to assign a number to our upset emotions helps us keep our lives in perspective.

With some professional help, Sylvia created a plan for building good days. We can do the same. We need to also remember to monitor ourselves so that we don't get too hungry, lonely, tired, or angry. When we experience these states, we can take immediate corrective action. We can learn to control our reactivity by breathing deeply and slowly. We can take mini-vacations that last five minutes or a day.

Yolanda, who runs a busy restaurant, has learned to schedule a massage on her day off. After that massage, she is able to relax and enjoy whatever happens over the weekend. By Monday morning she is ready to work again.

Lola handles property tax evaluations for the state and deals with angry people all week long. By Friday afternoon, she twitches with anxiety. She asks her husband to take her for a silent drive on pretty country roads. After an hour or two, they stop by a lake, watch the sun go down. The silence and the green landscape allow Lola to decompress.

Repetition gives us security, while variation provides zest. We want a balance between regular habits that are deeply satisfying and spontaneity with its freshness and excitement. We want a good strong comfort zone and we want to be able to push ourselves outside it on a regular basis.

Contrasts heighten our sensory awareness. For example, after we go sledding or cross-country skiing, it feels wonderful to sit by a fire and drink hot tea or cocoa. After swimming in cold water, a hot shower feels blissful. If we have been sitting at a desk all day, we can wake up our bodies and reenter the world of the senses by taking a long walk and preparing a meal of fresh vegetables. If we have experienced a week full of people, an evening alone is a blessing. If we have been lonely, we may be ready for a party.

"Subject change" is a good phrase for thinking about contrasts. A day feels fresher if every now and then we can say, "Subject change," and switch to doing something different. A vacation is a subject change and so is coming home. Working hard on a project, then stopping for a phone call, nap, or a cup of coffee is a subject change.

As we move from one activity to another, we can find ways to focus on the transition, to create the conditions for being present and positive about whatever happens next. For example, before we greet a visitor or pick up a telephone, we can spend a moment breathing and focusing on being present for the moment to come. This allows us to truly pay attention to whomever we are meeting.

Perhaps the most important factor in building a good day involves managing expectations. Globally, happiness correlates with reasonable expectations. Intuitively this makes sense—the higher our expectations are about anything—an upcoming meal, a reunion, or a vacation—the more likely we are to be disappointed. If we expect our days to be problem-free, we set ourselves up for disappointment and complaint. Much of life is solving problems.

Psychology researchers have found there are two primary types of people: minimizers, who keep their expectations low, and maximizers, who want every experience to be a little better than it is. The maximizers can pitch their tents in the best spots on a glorious June night but then notice a spider and consider their campout ruined. Minimizers tend to be satisfied with what they have. They settle for "good enough" experiences. On a camping trip when it is rainy and they forget the hot dogs, they are still likely to say they had fun. Fortunately, maximizers can teach themselves to tamp down expectations and correct their tendencies to allow small disappointments to color entire events. Over time, doing so will make them much happier.

With older women, everything comes with an asterisk. We can enjoy our lives if we acknowledge their intensity and poignancy and if we have reasonable expectations. My aunt Grace said, "I get what I want, but I know what to want."

A skill similar to maintaining reasonable expectations is keeping things in perspective. Thirty years ago, my husband and I lost a good friend to brain cancer and since then, when we start to get worked up, we tell each other, "This isn't brain cancer." When people lose their homes in tornadoes or hurricanes, we often hear the most resilient ones saying, "At least nobody died."

When times are tough, think short-term. Long-term, we are all going to die. But short-term, we can plan for happiness, one day at a time. If life is particularly rough, think in terms of the next ten minutes.

A variant of this idea is the importance of breaking complicated projects down into one step at a time. Suzuki music teachers know this strategy well. With small enough steps, children can learn to play symphonies. Similarly, we can break down a complicated process, such as changing residences, into small manageable steps. I like the one-hour-a-day rule for overwhelming tasks. If a job is overwhelming, I tell myself, just work on it for an hour today. Over time I will complete it.

The only real time is noticed time. Perhaps one of the best gifts we can give ourselves is to practice slowing down and doing one thing at a time. Almost all of us have trouble doing this. In fact, new research by Martin Seligman suggests that we humans are wired to think about the future, to anticipate, plan, and worry. As one of my friends put it, "I'm not sure I'll ever be present. There are so many layers between me and the moment."

Without an agenda, though, the world can be a bigger and more interesting place. Recently I gave my grandson a model Viking ship that required cutting and gluing for assembly. We worked on it for a few minutes, then Coltrane jumped up from the table, turned on his electric piano, and began to sing and dance.

For a while, I tried to lure him back to the ship. I even caught myself saying, "Nonna isn't going to build this ship by herself." Coltrane kept dancing. All of a sudden, I woke up to the moment. I started dancing and singing with Coltrane. I suggested words such as "thunder" and "mountain" to help him create new songs. We both laughed at his sillier songs. This experience was a joyful lesson in living in the moment.

Life becomes so much simpler when we realize we are in no hurry. We can learn when to toss our lists out the window and step into the moment. When our old cat jumps into our lap, we can stop writing our to-do list and snuggle with our purring friend. If we are reading a magazine and a child shows up who wants to bake cookies, we can find the measuring spoons, flour, and sugar. When a friend suggests a walk while we are cleaning the garage, we can say, "Yes, yes, yes."

Eloise knew what was important and was a world-class appreciator. Four years ago, when she lost her husband to a lung disease, she wondered if she would ever be happy again, but over time, she rebuilt her life. She possessed the attitude and skills she needed to lead a good life in spite of loss.

Her husband, Bill Kloefkorn, had been an English professor at Nebraska Wesleyan University and the Nebraska State Poet. He had a big personality and an equally large life. Eloise had known him since high school. She dealt with her grief and found a balm for her loneliness in meaningful work.

Recently, I visited Eloise at the assisted living community where she now lives. When she met me at the entrance, I was struck by how vibrant she looked. She was a small, trim woman with bright brown eyes. She proudly showed me around her new home.

We walked down its "Main Street," where there was a travel agency, bank, and drugstore. There was also a fountain with goldfish and a large light-filled cafeteria. She pointed to a trail outside the cafeteria and told me it connects to our city trail system.

We took the stairs to her third-floor apartment. She pointed outside to her favorite feature—a balcony overlooking green space. She said that her happiest times were sitting on this balcony, reading or watching birds and other wildlife.

We sat in her living room filled with pictures of Bill and also of ceramic pigs, which Bill loved. While Eloise made coffee, she told me that she was mostly healthy and still drives. She kept in good touch with her friends and extended family.

Eloise told me, "When Bill died, I didn't even think of moving, I was so filled with grief." She stayed in their home for three years. But last year, with winter coming and a major home repair job looming, she decided to move. One of her children hated to see her sell the house, but Eloise said, "Bill would want me to be where I am safe and happy."

She talked about missing Bill. She likes to visit a site she calls "Bill's rock." She sits by this rock and fills him in on what has been happening with the family.

Lincoln's Kloefkorn Elementary School was named for Bill. In fourth grade, the children spend the year studying Bill's life and work. Eloise said that she visits that school several times a week, and talks to the children about Bill. She tells them about what he was like, and she helps them memorize his poems. Eloise told me that the children always ask how Bill died and she tells them the truth. They also ask her if she will die. She tells them, "Everyone will die. It's important to be happy while we are alive."

Talking to a grandmother figure such as Eloise helped children open up about their emotions. Eloise said, "Some of the children tell me about their grandparents' deaths. I just sit by them and listen."

Eloise talked some about losing relatives and friends. In a notebook, she keeps a record of the deaths of her friends and acquaintances by date. "Everyone in here loses people regularly. But that doesn't stop us from having a good time," she reflected.

She sings in the choir at her new home. She is in the walk-a-mile club that walks the indoor track together after every meal. She joined an in-house book club. Eloise said she likes to be around people, but she also likes the freedom to be alone. She finds gossipers and complainers irritating, and she has learned to avoid them. She is often happy to just read in her room.

One of her closest friends is another widow whose husband also worked at Nebraska Wesleyan. The two of them grieved together and now they meet regularly for breakfast and outings.

Eloise is grateful to have such a pleasant place to live and such a good quality of life. Neither Bill nor she ever made a large salary, but they were frugal. "I'm grateful to have the finances to live in a place like this," she said. "Many of my friends are not so fortunate."

As I walked out, Eloise showed me pictures on her refrigerator that the elementary-school children had drawn for her. My favorite was of a beautiful pig, labeled "For my friend, Mrs. Kloefkorn."

Eloise possesses excellent navigational skills and she knows how to create a good day for herself. After the loss of Bill, she discovered ways to flourish. She moved to a place easy to maintain, filled with plenty of interesting people. She both sings in a choir and savors her solitude. She has utilized the healthy habits of a lifetime to keep her life in balance. Eloise possesses the vital skills of knowing what to look for in life and how to enjoy it when she finds it.

We will find what we look for. When we look for humor, beauty, or joy, we will discover them all around us. Eloise likes to look for evidence of love wherever she goes. If she sees a couple holding hands while they wait for a bus, or a silver-haired lady carrying an ice-cream cone into a hospital, or a young child earnestly playing a cello at a recital, she feels a ping of pleasure at further evidence of love in the universe.

Our consciousness is crafted by attention. Happiness requires us to make the choice to pay attention to this and not that. Horseback riders know that the horse will go in the direction the rider is looking. We can learn to look toward where we want to be.

Closing the day is a vital part of experiencing a good day. As we wait for sleep to come, it's soothing to reflect upon what happened during the day that we learned from, felt proud of, or enjoyed, and to reenvision our happiest moments. We can also pray or meditate—much more calming activities than worrying.

Last night I awoke around four a.m. after a nightmare that involved death, imprisonment, and children being mistreated. I was so agitated that I couldn't go back to sleep. I breathed deeply and slowly for a while.

I said a prayer for all those who were suffering, and then I decided to remember my grandparents' small home in Flagler, Colorado.

I had not been in their home in more than forty-five years, but I could still walk from room to room in my mind, remembering the pictures on my grandmother's dressing table, the card table in the living room where we played dominoes and checkers, the picture window in the dining room that looked out on the ash tree, and the kitchen with its small red table and my grandmother at the stove. I saw the jars of canned fruits in the root cellar. Soon, I could taste the small blue plums that she canned and recall the way her dishes were arranged in the kitchen cabinets. Remembering her porcelain cookie jar filled with oatmeal and molasses cookies, I drifted off to sleep.

Creating Community

"Develop skin as tough as a rhino's hide. You cannot take
anything personally. You cannot bear grudges. You must finish
the day's work when the day's work is done. Don't be easily
discouraged. Take defeat over and over, pick yourself up,
and go on." —Eleanor Roosevelt

"Empathy . . . is the most revolutionary emotion."
—Gloria Steinem

NORA AND ROGER have lived in a small suburban community most of their adult lives. When they retired, they decided to do something to help their town. After some conversation, they realized that the entire community was without a park. So, they organized a group of friends to change that. This was a long-term project that required raising money, finding affordable land central to key housing areas, and working through the bureaucracy to get permits. Four years later their group was planting trees, buying fountains and playground equipment, and setting up courts for bocce and pickleball.

Nora and Roger planted a gingko tree in honor of Nora's mother, who had died during the course of the project. They walked to the park every evening and greatly enjoyed seeing all the families picnicking. Long after Nora and Roger are gone, their suburb will have a place for children and adults to enjoy.

Action is the antidote to despair. It may or may not help the world, but it always helps us. Hope comes from engaging in a hopeful process, such as planting a community garden, donating time or money to good causes, or helping people in our polarized country respect and empathize with each other.

We older women are uniquely suited for community work. We have been accumulating skills for decades and have so many things we know how to do. Often we have lived in the same place for years and we know what the challenges are and how to work the system for the greater good. If we are lucky, we can be "connectors," people who connect people to each other and to resources.

We have the wisdom of our years, knowledge of the world, and the time to tackle complicated, long-term problems. We can develop relationships with people in power and access information. We can help children, younger adults, and older people. With a commitment to do this, we have agency. The belief in our own power creates power.

Even those of us who are interested in global issues often find that when it comes to making a difference, we can achieve the most in our local communities. That is where we have the most knowledge, influence, and passion. Whether we are interested in governance, education, social justice, or environmental issues, usually we can be most effective when we work close to home.

Lynne was in charge of group singing on a retreat I attended at Ghost Ranch. She was a lively leader with a beautiful voice. At the end of the retreat, I asked if I could interview her.

Lynne was married to a man whose wife had died and left him with five children. Mordecai was a lifelong activist and community organizer in Philadelphia. Lynne respected his work, but had been too busy raising his children to be deeply engaged herself. When the last child left home, Lynne became more involved. She felt the urgency of our ecological and global refugee crises. She developed a network called the Conscious Elders Network, which taps into older people's desire to work for good causes. People all around the country have joined this group.

Lynne feels that she is embracing herself as an elder. She likes the phrase "elderhood" to describe older adults who have taken responsibility to fix things. She's sixty-seven now and feels she has ten or fifteen years left to be actively involved in changing the world. She said, "These are my glory years. I am my freest and most empowered."

As she ages, she grows more reflective. "I have time to consider the big questions now," she explained. "My definition of successful aging is having loving relationships and a life of engagement and meaning."

Lynne said that she would like to face her own death with curiosity. She would like to feel that the world is a better place because she existed. She said, "It has been such a privilege and honor to be alive. As I grow older, I try not to focus on my regrets and failures, but rather to focus on what I've accomplished." Lynne feels that life itself is a garden that she wants to be working on until she is gone. She wants to add a little more color here, a little more depth here, and a spot of brightness wherever she can.

Every one of us has something to give to someone. Whatever our gifts, we can offer them. We can check in on an isolated neighbor in the next apartment or volunteer at the hospital. We can sort clothing for the homeless or work in a soup kitchen. We can teach Sunday school or serve on a board. We can pick up litter in a park or deliver Meals on Wheels. There is a job for each of us, no matter our talents or interests.

Many of the happiest women I know are activists. As I write this, I think of Nancy quoting from the Bible at a legislative hearing concerning fracking wastewater and I see Christy hosting fundraisers for young people running for office. When we do advocacy work we engage with people of all ages and points of view. We also continually learn more about the world. Author David Brooks wrote that joining a group that meets once a month produces the same amount of happiness in people as doubling their income does. I am not sure this would apply to our poorest citizens, but I can attest that membership in a good group is happiness-producing.

Activism is complicated. When we are victorious, we can feel jubilant, but losses, especially on critical issues, can bring us down. Furthermore, all activists need to set limits or we can become exhausted and burned out. A passionate person can find important work every hour of every day. I have friends who email me at midnight on a Saturday with new information about a climate issue or policy change. We should endeavor to keep our advocacy activities in balance. It is good to work and it is good to rest.

Sandy moved to Lincoln and immediately immersed herself in multiple volunteer projects. She was responsible and intelligent and much valued by all the groups she worked with. However, after about six months, she withdrew from everything. In her eagerness to be helpful, she had worn herself out. I am hoping that, after some time away, she will again become a strong advocate for good causes. Perhaps, next time around, she will be more protective of herself and thus be able to stay involved.

This cautionary tale applies to us all. We don't want to go overboard. If that means we only help others an hour a week, so be it. If we are someone who loves naps or being in bed by nine at night, we can find work that allows us to continue doing what we love. If we only want to work with animals, we can find a way to do that. One of the great joys of this life stage is we can learn to grant ourselves permission to rest and to savor our own lives. If we don't rest, we can burn out and decide that helping others isn't for us. That is a sad conclusion for us and for the world.

We all want to be helpful, but we don't want to waste time. We want to know relevant information, but not be burdened with a great deal of worry about things we are unlikely to impact. I distinguish between "actionable intelligence" and what I call "distractionable intelligence."

An example of actionable intelligence in Nebraska was the news that an enormous chicken-processing plant was applying for permits upriver from our community. This plant could compromise our air and water and put our health at risk. Citizens could act on this information and call our legislators or organize protests and community education sessions. On the other hand, in Nebraska, when we hear that the oceans are becoming more acidic or that the ice caps are melting, we feel helpless.

None of us has the responsibility to singlehandedly save the world, but we all can do our best given our circumstances. Usually doing our best means working with others. Groups are more effective than individuals at getting things done. Working with others allows us to share the challenges and find solace in our common burdens.

There is a place for us to be useful in every community. Whatever our passions, whatever our talents, we can find a group to help us improve the world. We can choose to work with people we like. None of us will persist in community work if it is made unpleasant by difficult group members.

It's easy to form a group. We can invite one person out for coffee and agree on a cause. Once we know what our goal is, we can ask others to join us. Our best bet is to ask people we know who have some kind of special knowledge or skills to contribute. Invitation-only groups allow us to work with people we can count on.

For the last eight years I've been involved in a group that formed to stop the Keystone XL pipeline in our state. Our group formed when a young guy named Brad, who was helping me prune trees, talked with me about his fears about global climate change. I felt the same way he did. We agreed to ask a few of our friends to come to a dinner at my house the next week and talk over what we could do. All these years later, we are still going strong. We work on issues besides the Keystone XL, such as clean energy, promoting local foods, educating our state about climate change, and protecting our water supply.

Our group has achieved a great deal including, at least until now, helping stop the KXL from being built. We have also encouraged environmentalists to run for public office and raised awareness of environmental issues in our citizens and our legislature. But one of our main achievements is lifting the hearts and minds of group members. We emphasize fun and caring. We meet once a month for potlucks in private homes. We have wine and delicious homemade meals. Our meetings are as much like parties as serious discussions can be. Both our mission and our fun together have kept the group going across the years.

Of course, our group has its share of rather tedious tasks. But we try to make them fun and we support each other when we are doing the difficult work that sometimes must be done. We have worked together year after year on projects we believe to be vitally important. We exchange information about events and we plan actions. Our group's youngest member is toddler Bob, who started attending when he was a newborn. Mostly our members are either in their twenties and early thirties or over sixty-five. The demographic in between those ages tends to be busy raising children and making a living.

Working together is a great deal of fun. We older women host the meetings and cook simple meals. We tend to be the ones with connections, resources, and the understanding of how things work locally. Younger people are high-energy and provide physical labor and social media expertise. Many of our younger members are artists and involved with the music community, so it is easy to plan awareness-raising educational forums, festivals, and concerts. We have so much to teach each other.

For a while we older women were baking apple pies to give as awards to local politicians who behaved in ways that protected the environment. Whenever we did this, we called a press conference so that the person being honored would be in the newspaper with a good visual. Who doesn't like a free home-baked apple pie?

Instead of feeling hopeless, sad, or angry at the problems we saw in the world, we built a group. And we have grown to care for each other. Martin Luther King Jr. described working for the common good with others as participating in a beloved community. That is what our group feels like by now.

We don't all need to form groups. We can join existing groups or sign up for some kind of community service. Several of the women in my neighborhood work together at polling stations. Another group of friends is in a small choir that sings at nursing homes. The important thing is knowing our own strengths and talents and employing them in service to our communities.

I met with three community leaders at our local African American community center, called the Malone Center. Ella and Corinne were in their late sixties and Sharon was seventy-five. Corinne was a plump and relaxed woman dressed in blue jeans and a sweatshirt. Sharon wore a printed dress and had her makeup and hair carefully arranged. Ella, frail and soft-spoken, sat between them and softly encouraged the conversation with her nods and her pats on her friends' arms.

Corinne introduced herself as a deeply religious person. Before her father died, he recommended she join a church. He wanted her to have a place in a loving community. She had never considered this before, but she took his advice. She is grateful for her decision. She now has people she feels safe with, who she laughs with, and who will take care of her. Her most important goal is developing a closer relationship to God.

Ella is a cancer survivor who works hard to stay healthy. She is a life-long learner and takes community college classes in African American history. She volunteers for the Red Cross and a program that mentors at-risk youth. In her free time, she walks around her neighborhood; if she sees children behaving inappropriately, or hears them swearing, she encourages them to be better behaved. At first the kids seemed insulted, but now they like her and give her respect. She said, "I don't see the rude behavior I used to see."

Sharon is a lifelong activist. She told me that she likes to help people of all races. She worked at a human services agency most of her life, and now runs support groups for domestic violence survivors and recent parolees. She teaches group members to stand up for themselves but also to be responsible adults engaged with the community.

Sharon, Ella, and Corinne are constantly asked to do more. They want to help, but they also want to enjoy their years in this life stage. They are judicious in what work they agree to do. Ella has learned to say, "I'll think about it." All of them have a rule not to accept any requests for help without pondering it for a day. They stop work at sunset and take Sundays off. "Even God didn't work on Sundays," Corinne said.

They all have their pleasures. Both Corinne and Sharon like to drive in the country to relax. Sharon enjoys dancing on Saturday evenings. Ella loves to read and listen to music. They are all Scrabble and card players.

The three women had lived in an area historically populated by African Americans called the Malone neighborhood. They agreed that the area had changed greatly. For most of their lives it was a strong and vibrant community, where people knew each other and knew what was happening on the streets. Sharon laughed and said, "We couldn't do anything wrong because everybody paid attention."

In the past, many adults helped their community members. Corinne's mother assisted high school students with college and financial aid applications. Older people sat on porches and kept an eye on things. The Malone Center was packed every day with families who came together for activities. Ella said that community leaders were visible, vocal, and inspiring.

However, over the last fifteen years, things have changed. The university wanted to expand into the neighborhood; they bought land and many buildings and houses were condemned. The community was shattered and many traditions disappeared. The women said that they did not feel angry about this; they felt sad. They remembered when the people in their area were close to each other and when families were healthier.

The women agreed that historically, African Americans have been more respectful of older women than white Americans have been. Even now, African Americans are unlikely to put older relatives in nursing homes. But they sadly agreed that older women are not respected the way they used to be. Sharon said that younger parents are not teaching their children to honor their elders. They all believed that children today watch too much television and play too many video games.

The women were discouraged by this, but also eager to take responsibility to improve the situation. Sharon said, "I want to work until the day I die."

"Well I do, too, but I want easy work," Ella said, laughing. "I just want to love people."

"I try to follow the Golden Rule," Corinne said. "That's a lot of work."

All three women sat on their porches when the weather was pleasant. They greeted their neighbors and visited with young moms about their children. They knew the names of the people and dogs on their street, and they kept an eye on things. Corinne laughed as she said, "We can do plenty of good work from our front porches."

One of our best models for how to act together for the common good is offered by Native American culture. Many native peoples share traditions that involve a deep sense of connection with all living beings and with Mother Earth. They have great respect for the history and the traditions of their people. They think in long timelines. Decisions are made with a view to future generations, including generations of plants and animals.

I spent a morning talking to an Omaha tribal member about her work for future generations. I had met Renée at a water blessing ceremony at Spring Creek Prairie. She was dressed in traditional clothing and chanting by a small pond. She was a tall, stately woman with long black hair and an open, kind face.

Two weeks later, I visited her home for a conversation. Native American art blanketed her walls and a table displayed eagle feathers and braided sweetgrass. She was a soft-spoken woman with a great sense of mission.

When I asked her what tribe she was from, she answered with a story that took two hours to tell. It began when her people moved with the Ojibway from Quebec to the Missouri River, and it ended with her current work as a warrior, water protector, community healer, and linguist.

Renée never spoke about herself as an individual, but rather as a tribal member. She conceptualized events as one small part of a long timeline. For example, she sees the fight against the Dakota Access Pipeline near Standing Rock as part of native peoples' continuous struggle to protect their land, water, and treaty rights.

She explained that during the 1700s, the Omaha were a prosperous and populous people. They controlled the Missouri River from Missouri into South Dakota. Then in 1804 they lost many of their tribe to smallpox.

This devastation destroyed the cultural history of the tribe. Many of the storytellers, medicine women, spiritual leaders, and master crafts-people perished in this plague. By the time French fur traders arrived, the culture was already in shambles.

Renée is a descendant of an Omaha chief's daughter who was married to a French trader. Traders married into tribes to cement their relationships with tribal leaders. Also, the new wives often spoke several local languages and could be translators.

Renée's parents were activists in the Lincoln community and part of the American Indian Movement. Dennis Banks, Russell Means, and many other leaders came to dinner at her family's house. When she was a girl, her parents took her to Wounded Knee. She told me, "From the time I was young I felt I would do important work. I was not meant for small jobs."

Even as a girl, she has been a student of culture. She learned about her tribe at the annual solstice and equinox gatherings. At these events, she noticed that people referred to ancient ceremonies but they didn't know how to perform them. She decided that she would study the tribe's history and ceremonies and then teach them to others.

When she was eighteen, Renée moved from Lincoln onto the Omaha Reservation near Macy. At first, she was not used to reservation ways, but eventually she loved it. She felt at home there. After she received a college degree, she taught the Omaha children about their history, ceremonies, and language.

Renée married a man from the Lakota Sioux tribe. She became a designated water protector. She participated in sweat lodge ceremonies and received her first eagle plume. Eventually, she became an official warrior of the tribe. She now leads water ceremonies and vision quests for teenagers. She created a storytelling project. Renée told me, "When I work, energy shoots through my body. I know I am working on sacred ground."

All the women in this chapter have found ways to be connected and useful. They are happy elders who wake up with a sense of purpose that money can't buy. They have found their antidote to despair. When we organize and work together, we have the power to change the world. Whoever we are, wherever we are, we are needed. When we act for the good, we move into our own power and into more authentic and connected lives.

CHAPTER 12

Crafting Resplendent Narratives

"A few stories are sinking ships, and many of us go down with these ships even when the lifeboats are bobbing all around us . . . We think we tell stories, but stories often tell us, tell us to love or to hate, to see or to be blind. Often, too often, stories saddle us, ride us, whip us onward, tell us what to do and we do it without questioning." —Rebecca Solnit

"It is memory that provides the heart with impetus, fuels the brain, and propels the corn plant from seed to fruit." —Joy Harjo

SYLVIA IN AUSTIN has learned that she is in control not of life, but of the story about her life. She chuckles when she thinks of her grandchildren doing hip-hop dances in her kitchen to Christmas music or selling lemonade in their front yard to the crowds at South by Southwest. She is grateful she has such joy-producers in her life. She even believes that, as the grandchildren work their magic on him, Lewis may feel happy again. She values herself as a person who does her duty to the best of her ability. Even her wayward, addicted daughter may someday return home. Sylvia has a bed for her.

We can't change our pasts, but we can still change our stories. It isn't just long histories that influence our lives; it's also the narratives we tell ourselves about that history. Stories allow us to make sense of our lives, resolve our omnipresent contradictions, and understand ourselves and other people. They give us the context for comprehending the flow of life that constantly surrounds us.

We don't apprehend the world, but rather we construct it with our senses, our memories, and our ways of framing experience.

Sometimes, stories change abruptly. Many of us know someone who was supposedly "happily married" until her divorce. Then, overnight, the decent, "good-enough" spouse morphs into a selfish, narcissistic oaf. At one time or another, most of us have experienced a kind of story-whiplash as we tried to reconcile our memories with a friend's new story. On the other hand, most of us gradually change our story with time.

Functional stories are based on reality and include, at some level, everything that has happened to us—our mistakes, regrets, and traumas, but also our victories, joys, and moments of strength. We acknowledge our own points of view, but recognize that others see things differently.

Basing our stories on reality is much harder than it sounds. None of us does this completely. Facts turn out to be elusive. We assume a great deal and take too much for granted. We believe our own fantasies, run toward comforting illusions, and avoid unpleasant certainties. Or we hand-select woes to make problem-saturated stories and stew in our grief.

When our stories make us feel sad, isolated, and powerless, we can craft a better story, not at the expense of truth, but rather in the service of cheerfulness and gratitude.

There are merciful and positive ways to think about others and ourselves. Whole chunks of story can be reenvisioned. We can remember our history of resilient responses. We can compose narratives that serve us. Even our most painful experiences can be revisited. We can ask, "How did that make me stronger?" "What did I learn from that experience?" "What am I proud of when I look back on that day?"

We can slowly train ourselves to think in stories that allow us to flourish. We hone our skills in perspective taking, emotional processing, and reframing. Stories of joy, kindness, and courage empower us in ways that the culturally stereotyped narrative never does.

• • •

WILLOW WAS ABLE to cope with Saul's Parkinson's and her retirement by crafting a new story. She told herself, "I have a new life now and new priorities." She felt a tenderness and a great rush of loyalty toward Saul. Her identity shifted from her professional work to her capacities to care for Saul and herself through hard times. She awoke thinking, "What would make us happy today?"

Her priority was creating good moments for the two of them. She fixed his favorite meals, gave him back rubs, and told him jokes when she helped him shower. One day, he laughed so hard he said, "Cut that out or I'm going to fall down." That made them laugh some more.

They lay in bed reading the newspaper or playing gin rummy. This low-key time turned out to be surprisingly fun for Willow. As Saul's health situation worsened, he became more jovial and philosophical. Every day, she loved him more.

Like Willow, we all can honor our pain and then move toward something more joyful. We can focus on our resilience and remember our joys or sorrows. We can craft stories that tell us we are loved, strong, resilient, respected, worthy, generous, forgiven, and happy. We all have such stories, if only we can uncover them.

"I am saved" or redemption stories are often positive. Alcoholics Anonymous and Narcotics Anonymous help people create redemption stories and so do evangelical churches where people are "born again." Even renewing our wedding vows can be a redemption story. This ceremony can imply that we were certain people long ago and now we are different people committing to a new person for a new life.

Reconciliation stories abound. The Prodigal Son is such a story but there are many mother and prodigal daughter stories too. Reconciliation stories consider sisters who reunite, friends who find the vehicles of mercy to forgive, and other stories about making peace and moving joyfully into the future. Many people have been enormously heartened by being able to tell themselves, "Somebody needs me."

To rewrite our story, we need effort and imagination. We can access imagination by journaling, painting, music, or art. One of my favorite things about writing is that I get to tell a second story about whatever happens to me. And, in this second story, I can shape events in ways that are more beautiful and happiness-producing. Indeed, what is all art, if not an attempt to tell a better story?

Some of our stories bring out the best in us, whereas others induce despair, fear, or anger. We can ask ourselves questions that remind us of our kindness, hard work, and strength over the years. We can explore our uncelebrated virtues and our survival skills.

When we consider others' viewpoints, our narratives become more clear, complex, and useful. Friends can listen to our woes and then remind us of other stories that we have told them. When we are blue, it helps to be reminded that we have been through tough times before and that we rescued ourselves. Partners often help with this. My friend Linda wrote a short summary of her adult life for her fiftieth high school reunion. When her husband read it, he said, "You only described your losses and failures. Why don't you tell about your success at work and your new hobby—horseback riding?"

When Emma is overscheduled and frantic because of too many commitments, her Rock of Gibraltar, Chris, will often hug her and use humor to help her put things in perspective. When she tells him that Alice is driving her crazy, he will invariably respond with "That's not a drive, that's a short putt." They will laugh and Emma will feel better. If nothing else, she knows that her situation is not so grim they can't joke about it.

Kestrel had some trouble crafting a new narrative. She had always protected herself with thorns and quills. When that didn't work, she medicated her pain with alcohol. She felt lonely but safe in her walled-off state.

The summer her mother got cancer, Kestrel's old story stopped working. She didn't feel safe and she could no longer numb her fear with booze. Suddenly she felt a need for human comfort and closeness.

She realized that her anger had kept her emotionally protected at great cost. She'd missed the possibility of connection and even love. Loving her mother wasn't a great challenge, but trusting Becca with her heart felt scary as could be, almost scarier than her father's anger.

As Kestrel teeter-tottered between need and fear, Becca listened and respected her boundaries. Then one night, when Becca and Kestrel were talking on the phone, Kestrel said, "Let's go steady when I come back."

They both laughed. Becca said, "You've got a deal."

Suddenly Kestrel had a new story: "I've got a girlfriend."

• • •

CEREMONIES AND EVENTS give us opportunities to formulate new stories. We older women often have multiple ways to revisit stories. We can attend class reunions, family weddings, and birthday and anniversary celebrations. Even funerals and memorial services are reunions of those people who cared for a particular person.

Many of us find these occasions allow us to reframe our narratives. When we talk to others about their memories of our shared past, we realize how many vantage points there are on one particular time. We can ask, "What do you remember about my family?" "What do you recall about me as a girl?" or "How do you remember eighth grade?"

We can plan and enact rituals that signal we are moving into a different story. Every year in January, my daughter-in-law and I drive to a retreat center to be together in a way that leads us from the story of one year to the story of the next. We spend our time reading, in silence, or talking about the year that passed and the year that we hope to make happen. Our discussions allow us to consciously craft healing stories. Some people can turn doing their laundry into a fascinating narrative while others can make a trip to Antarctica seem boring. The difference is emotion and motive. "The king died; the queen died" is a statement of fact. "The king died; the queen died of grief" is a story. Stories are always an interpretation of facts.

With age, we can become more skillful at telling heartening stories. For example, when a friend is brusque with us, we are likely to think, "She's having a bad day." When we were younger, we might have thought,

"She doesn't like me anymore." This is because most of us have learned not to take things personally. Almost everything that happens in the universe is not about us.

As a therapist, I tried to help clients create better stories. I asked questions such as, "When have you been courageous or stronger than you thought you could be?" "What would your life look like if you were happy and satisfied?"

When I have worked with trauma victims, I inquired, "When you look back at the dreadful situation, what were you able to do that you felt proud of?" This question elicited answers such as "When I was being raped I fought back. And afterward, I called the police." Or "No matter how lost I felt on my journey to America, I tried to be kind to people I met along the way."

Over the years, I have seen clients who had almost no stories to tell. They didn't remember their childhoods and they did not recollect experiences as they went about their adult lives. I encouraged them to talk to anyone who remembered them as a child or young adult and ask them for stories and information. I suggested they visit places they had lived or gone to school. Evoking memories through the senses helps us with reconstructions.

When clients focused on positive sensory memories, they often pictured their summer vacation on a beach or the aroma of their grandmother's cooking or the sound of music on a city street. These memories helped them put their pain from the past in perspective. They remembered they had been happy and that people had loved them.

Every sense is evocative. Certain sensations may bring us pain and sorrow, but others may evoke joy. Foods often spark our memories. When I taste what my aunts used to cook, I am tasting time. Or we can simply remember foods. I haven't cooked chipped beef on toast for my children's breakfast in thirty years, but I can taste it now as I write this. I can see our tiny kitchen with its cracked red linoleum floor, and I can see the faces of my young children as they eagerly lapped up gravy. That memory makes me smile.

When I recently visited my son's high school and walked past the swimming pool where he became a state champion, I could picture him, with his goggles and blue swimsuit on the starting block, in position for the race buzzer. I could smell the chlorine in the air and remember the adrenaline of excitement from thirty years ago. I could hear the shouts of the parents and his teammates as Zeke finished a race.

Perhaps the most evocative of all the senses is auditory, especially if it's a musical memory. We remember music from both sad and happy periods of our lives, but if we focus on the music from our happy times we will recall events that make us smile. Ellen Langer's research demonstrates that when people hear the music of their youth, not only do musical memories return, but many other memories as well. Her research also shows that we can improve our health and mental health by listening to music from times when we were happy.

Sometimes stories stick around way beyond their "sell-by date." If we experienced trauma as children, we likely learned to deal with our pain in unhelpful ways. We denied it, buried it, or acted it out with others. We numbed or injured ourselves, or decided not to trust other people. We may still be fighting a lifelong struggle with anxiety, depression, anger, or regret. No matter how high quality our lives are, we may feel unable to see ourselves as anything but victims.

I had the chance to rethink an old story when Jim and I attended the Rocky Mountain Folks Festival. We'd had a summer that involved caring for grandchildren and helping my sister through three hospital stays, a stint in rehab, and various arrangements for in-home nursing and physical therapy. Arriving in Colorado, with the children happily ensconced in daycare and my sister temporarily okay, I felt carefree for the first time in many months.

Jim and I had our usual fun. We dined at an Italian restaurant on Pearl Street. At our cabin, I slept on an outdoor porch that abuts the Flatiron Mountains and fell asleep looking at stars. Friday we attended the festival in all its folksy glory. Saturday, I decided to have one day in which I did whatever I felt like doing.

Jim dropped me off at Pearl Street late that morning and headed on to the festival. I walked to one of my favorite places, the Boulder Book Store, and I lost myself in books. Later, I ambled next door to a café with outdoor dining and ordered sushi and a glass of wine. I watched people walk by. I savored each bite of fish and each sip of wine. After an hour or so, I began the slow climb back to our room. By now it was hot, and I was grateful I had a water bottle. On my way, I turned into the Columbia Cemetery, an old graveyard that Jim and I had driven by for years. We'd always been too busy to stop, but this afternoon I had time.

I wandered about, looking at the old settlers' graves, some dating back to the 1840s. I looked for the tombstones of women and children and read the crumbled old inscriptions, many of which carried the agony of the moment in which they were conceived. Rosa Peterman, who had died at age ten on May 6, 1881, had a small white stone that depicted a girl diving and the words "Our Rosa." Another stone memorialized two brothers, Larry, aged four years, three months, and twenty days, and Roy, aged six months, twenty days, who died within six days of each other in January of 1880. Their crumbling gravestone featured two small doves flying away together.

In cemeteries, the same thought always arises for me: "They come and they go. We come and we go." This thought gives me a sense of peace.

I lay down on the grass between graves and looked at the sky. I thought of a Japanese word that a friend had taught me. "Komorebi" describes the way sunlight filters through leaves. My first memory, when I was a small child lying on a quilt on the grass, is of sunlight dancing in the leaves at the top of a tree. All of my life I have looked for that pattern of sparkling light and shadow. That afternoon in the old cemetery, the sunlight sparkled and faded in the branches of the elms and maples above me. Beyond, the sky was Rocky Mountain blue dappled with clouds gathering for a late-afternoon thunderstorm.

I arrived at our little cabin mid-afternoon and read until bedtime. I stopped occasionally to munch on fresh figs and peaches, and I moved from the front porch to the back porch as the sun moved across the sky. I can't remember a day when I was so happy.

The next day I realized that what I had done was much larger than the sum of its parts. I had experienced something I don't recall ever experiencing, although maybe I had in college or just afterward, before I was pregnant with my now-forty-four-year-old son, Zeke. I enjoyed a day when I did whatever I wanted all day long. And, I was moving slowly and quietly enough to be genuinely contemplative. From this solitude, I began to craft a new story.

My most common story is that someone needs me and I must rescue him/her. This story has led me to make many impulsive offers to help. No doubt, sometimes no help is needed. And many times, I have neither the time nor the talents nor the inclination to help.

On further reflection, I realized that I often become my own worst enemy, constantly signing myself up for combat duty when I really want to stay home, pet my cat, and read a book. Or, I harm myself when I truly want to see a friend, but make no time for it because I am too busy meeting the real or imagined needs of others.

This story of being a rescuer comes from a long time ago, when I was a needy little girl who could only feel safe if I reassured myself that I was helpful. I don't judge that little girl. Her story was, I still believe, quite close to reality. Furthermore, as an identity, being a good helper isn't the worst choice. That story led me to a life of satisfying work. But now I realized I could choose whether or not to continue that "little Mary" story.

I felt a little overwhelmed at the thought of making major life changes. Perhaps it was best to accept who I am. Yet a part of me was crying "uncle" at the thought of a lifetime of continuous helpful behavior. What if I just stopped trying to be heroic every day of my life? What if I could lose my constant vigilance about the needs of others, a habit I acquired when I was a big sister in a family with mostly absent parents? Could I lose this no longer functional habit and simply be present? Could I enter situations with no expectations about how others should be? For a few minutes at a time, could I lead a non-purpose-driven life?

Of course, these questions led to new stories of vacations, retreats and writing workshops, or of waking up rested and leisurely deciding how to spend a day. I smiled at these thoughts. That one day in Colorado showed me how much fun caring for myself could be.

With intention, perhaps I can live within this more self-cherishing story. Not all the time, of course. My driven need to save the world all by myself will return. Even writing books comes from my deep need to be helpful, but I love the writing process, and actually, if I don't overdo it, I enjoy making people feel loved, safe, and comfortable. But maybe I can be more self-protective when I choose to be. Perhaps I did learn to give myself a little wiggle room.

Mary Oliver said, "It was a very bad childhood for everybody, every member of the household, not just myself, I think. And I escaped it, barely. With years of trouble." Especially for women who were sexually, physically, or emotionally abused, inner scars continue to sting. Some of us had parents who were alcoholics, mentally ill, or physically or emotionally unavailable to us. Even if we are reasonably content now, we still carry that heritage.

When we experience a sad event, it is natural to react to it with pain. The first arrow is the event. Our prolonged reactions to the event are the second arrows. It is natural to need time to recover. But we make it harder for ourselves when we second-guess ourselves and feel guilty or ashamed. Instead, we can work with and modify these emotions from the second arrow. We can have both the courage to accept our suffering and the skills to move beyond it. We can pardon ourselves and all those around us.

This may be the most important thing—that we learn to grant ourselves mercy. That we forgive ourselves, that we accept our pain, mistakes, and vulnerability, and somehow manage to love ourselves and our own lives. Most of us do make progress in this area; all of us can make more. And it is only when we grant ourselves mercy that we can extend this mercy to others.

A friend told me about an artist who walked along the beaches gathering up the broken wood from houses and stores destroyed in Hurricane Sandy. Many of the pieces were small and jagged. She took these pieces of wood and formed them into beautiful wooden quilt-style works of art that now hang in galleries and private homes. That is a perfect metaphor for what we can do with wreckage.

The tragic events of our lives may never cease causing sorrow. Remembering our departed friends and family members can continue to fill us with heartache. Birthdays, holidays, and anniversaries can stay dark and lonely. If we have been traumatized in the past, we may always experience its echoes. But with motivation and skills even the greatest sorrows abate with time.

Meanwhile, some minor tragedies can become farcical. Many of us have a vacation-from-hell story that morphs into our favorite laugh-out-loud story to tell at parties. Or we have most-embarrassing-moment stories that now are our old standbys when we want to make others laugh. Misery loves company and, when we laugh together at our failings and our goof-ups, we can sometimes turn tragedy into comedy.

Good stories build good lives. When we are lonely we can remember our good times with loved ones, a blazing sunset, or our sixtieth birthday dinner when everyone told us precisely what they loved about us. When we reexamine our stories with a focus on clarity, acceptance, and resilience, we grow in confidence and joy. Our stories, if carefully considered, allow us to heal from the pain of the past and live vibrantly in the present.

We could define wisdom as the capacity to skillfully select our narratives. When we do this, we experience our lives as filled with meaning. Every present-day event resonates with the decades of past events. We can be grateful for everything that led us to the moment we are inhabiting. This is how life becomes sacred. It is hallowed by story.

CHAPTER 13

Anchoring in Gratitude

"There was in all living things something limpid and joyous—
like the wet, morning call of the birds, flying up through the
unstained atmosphere." —Willa Cather

"Give thanks for unknown blessings that are already on their
way." —Native American prayer

IN HIGH SCHOOL, I struggled through Boris Pasternak's famous novel *Doctor Zhivago*. This book had an enormous cast of characters and the long Russian names seemed impossible to keep straight. But I took notes on the names and nicknames and eventually *Doctor Zhivago* amazed me. I underlined parts of almost every page and wrote down countless quotes to memorize.

These last few years, I've been rereading all my favorite classics, most of which I read decades ago. When I reread Pasternak's book last year, I understood that it had shaped the way I have lived.

Dr. Zhivago was a good man in a terrible time and place. He tried to be kind to everyone and offer hope to others regardless of circumstance. He felt great passion and love for the world, especially the world of family, books, and nature. He was swept up by swells of gratitude for whatever kindness or grace was offered to him. But most important, in terms of his influence on me, he always was on a search for beauty.

When he was crammed into a freezing train car, hungry and exhausted, returning home from the front during World War I, he focused on the beautiful scent of linden tree blossoms. At the end, as he rode slowly across Moscow to a doctor's appointment, he suffered a heart attack. He kept his attention on the shimmering violet dress of a woman walking on the sidewalk.

I learned from Pasternak that we can always create a moment in which we are flooded by beauty and that the more desperate the times, the more important it is that we seek this kind of moment. That knowledge has saved me over and over again and become an important part of who I am. It is perhaps my best coping tool.

As we age, we tend to improve our gratitude skills. Through trial and error learning, we know that if we focus on the good and positive, we see ourselves as lucky. Whereas, when we focus on grievances, past pains, regrets, and disappointments, we can make ourselves feel unlucky and miserable. Also, we are likely to have experienced sad events that propelled us toward gratitude as a means of psychic survival.

Gratitude is a life skill that can be improved with practice. Even during the toughest trials, we can learn to find things to enjoy and appreciate. I don't mean to imply that we can manage to be grateful every moment. That would be an unrealistic demand on ourselves. Feeling grateful is not a moral injunction, but rather, a healthy habit that we can learn to employ with greater frequency.

• • •

WE CAN'T ALWAYS rise to the occasion. One morning, Emma woke with a bad flu and an eye infection. Outside a dense fog covered her garden and the trees beyond. She thought, "I'm in the same dense fog that I see outside."

Chris came in to see if she was okay and she moaned, "No, no, no."

He offered to rub her back or make her some hot cider and she shook her head. He asked if she wanted him to stay home from work and she said, "Just leave me alone. It hurts to talk." He tried to kiss her goodbye but she waved him away.

Everything hurt and Emma could hardly think. She felt so sick that she stupidly wished she could die. That morning the whole world was the color of cement.

Emma wisely gave herself a day off from feeling grateful and kind-hearted and just lay around moaning. But the next morning, when she felt a little better, she pushed herself to remember what was good in her life. When Chris brought her tea, she appreciated its warmth and minty flavor. She gave him a kiss, nibbled on his ear, and, when he laughed, she laughed too.

• • •

DR. ROBERT EMMONS at the University of California, Davis, worked with transplant patients. In his study, two groups were asked to record their feelings about life. One group was instructed to add a daily list of five things or people they were grateful for. After twenty-one days, the gratitude list group had improved their scores on measures of positive adjustment and well-being. Both of these measures had declined for people who had not been asked to keep track of what they were grateful for.

Gratitude doesn't correlate with circumstance. In fact, it's been my experience that women with the worst luck tend to have the strongest gratitude skills. Muriel's mother is an example of this.

Muriel flew across the country to be with her mother as she lay dying in an ICU. Her mother slept almost all the time, but she wasn't in pain. Her breathing was labored and she could no longer eat or drink on her own. Most days Muriel simply sat holding her mother's hand and thinking about her mother's long sad history.

Her mother had been orphaned young and worked as a live-in house-keeper in her early teens. She later married an abusive man who abandoned her after their third child was born. With only an eighth-grade education, she earned her living cleaning hotel rooms and cooking for greasy spoon restaurants.

Muriel wished she'd had time and money to take her mother on a beach vacation. She tried unsuccessfully to remember one luxury her mother had ever enjoyed. All she could recall was her own dance recitals from fifty years ago. Her mother had loved attending those. Just then her mother woke with a start. She put her hands on either side of Muriel's face and pulled her in close—eye to eye. She told Muriel, "I have had a wonderful life. Remember that."

Her mother fell back onto the pillow asleep and, by the next morning, she was gone. Muriel realized her mother condensed everything she knew about life in that one sentence. She determined that she would hold it in her heart and work to become more grateful.

Many women I know actively cultivate gratitude. Margie sends her friends frequent emails in which her entire topic is what she has enjoyed and appreciated that day. Gretchen keeps a gratitude journal and writes down that which delights her. Some of us challenge each other to have the longest gratitude lists at the end of the day.

We can remind ourselves every morning that we have the gift of life and that we can attend to that which is loving, touching, or beautiful.

We can say grace before meals, just to thank the universe for giving us our bread and fruit.

My former editor Jane feels grateful whenever she walks into an art gallery. The work is sacred to her. It reminds her of the best that we humans offer each other. Birdsong is my temple bell. I try to remember when I hear birds singing to breathe deeply and appreciate what is around me.

When we can appreciate the smallest of gifts, we are wise women. The great ecstatic Benedictine abbess Hildegard of Bingen was said to be so grateful for the gift of a sardine that she wept.

Ironically, tragedy often catapults people toward gratitude whereas constant good fortune can actually make it hard to feel grateful. Privileged people may habituate to a comfortable, easy life. Small problems engender big complaints. For example, "Oh no, my flight to Paris has been changed and I now have a four-hour layover in Chicago" or "The landscaper can't come until next week and nothing will look right for our party."

However, when we lose a beloved, our salvation is to remember with gratitude the joys of that relationship. We feel grateful, not in spite of problems, but because of them. For example, my friend Jan was telling me how much she missed her distant grandchildren. Then she stopped herself and sighed. She shook off her pain mid-sentence by saying, "Life is so complicated, but so damn good."

At a musical event at a Lutheran church, I watched an elderly woman in an electric mobility scooter. She had a full-body brace and wore a purple shirt, flowery print skirt, and white socks. In spite of her obvious hardships, she was grinning as she swayed and danced in her chair while singing loudly, "You Are My Sunshine."

My recently widowed neighbor actively sought out joy and gratitude by visiting a pet store. She would stand and watch the baby ferrets play, then enjoy the soothing movements of multicolored tropical fish. Sometimes she held a kitten that was awaiting adoption. By the time she left the pet store she always felt happy to be alive in such a sweet world.

Recognizing our own contentment is an undervalued skill. Intense passion and excitement grab our attention, but contentment whispers in ways we may not notice. In fact, contentment is a basic building block of a happy life. When we are content, we can say, "Notice this. This is good."

Vicki Robin wrote, "We need to slow people down to the speed of wisdom." "Slow down," admonishes my brother Jake. He says, "The slower you travel the more you see. When you give up speed, you open up time."

I attended a silent retreat where we chewed each bite at least thirty times before swallowing. That weekend, chewing was such hard work that I left the table hungry. However, I found myself loving the rather bland food of the monastery. Finally, I had time to notice and appreciate every good flavor. I had always hated oatmeal but I found myself looking forward to my morning bowl of oats and thinking, "Who knew oatmeal could be so nutty and filled with flavor?"

From this retreat I learned that doing things slowly and paying attention makes them much more enjoyable. Time expands, the senses are awakened, and everything feels more spacious and free. Ever since then, when I eat a piece of chocolate or drink a cup of good coffee, I try to notice how much I like it.

All of us can find ourselves in "airplane mode," just floating along inattentive to everything around us. But if we learn the skill of waking ourselves up and savoring life, the present can be a great joy.

Yesterday, I attended the memorial service of an old friend. Later I worked in my garden, where all the rosebushes were in glorious bloom. In my prairie flower bed, the red poppies saluted. I examined golf ball–size tomatoes and picked basil for pesto. And, just as the sun set, a meadowlark sang from the top of our masthead tree. The last of the sun's rays illuminated its yellow breast as it called out, "We are alive. Be grateful."

Sally has experienced a more difficult life than most of us. She comes from a complicated family with more than her share of poverty, loss, and health problems. She manages chronic pain and she is frequently seriously ill. Yet she exudes gratitude.

The most cheerful people I've ever known were the ones with the greatest hardships. I remember Alma from my book *Another Country*. She was caring for her sixty-year-old daughter, who had been profoundly brain-damaged at birth and who never learned to walk, talk, or feed herself. Alma was the only person I ever met who was brave enough to put a whoopee cushion under me and to cackle with amusement when I tooted and blushed. She often had parties at her place because her daughter couldn't leave home and she had so many visitors that it was hard to fit in my interviews. I always left her home feeling better. She could make me laugh when no one else could.

When I arrived for an interview, Sally greeted me at the screen door in her wheelchair. She gave me a big hug and invited me into her kitchen for tea. She has curly black hair, freckles, and a warm smile. Because both her arms are weak, I poured the tea and carried the pot to the table. She told me she was excited for our interview. She said, "Getting old is such a freaking privilege!"

Sally has a small older house on a tree-lined street. Her home is filled with books, art, and music. She plays soul music on her radio and keeps a James Beard cookbook and the *Colorado Review* on her kitchen table. We drank our tea out of old china cups, with antique silver cream and sugar holders nearby. Sally had just baked bread, which she served with Irish butter. She winked and said, "I can afford the luxury of Irish butter."

Her son, Sean, is currently in Colorado helping a progressive candidate run for the Senate. Sean is a burly, talkative guy who has worked as a prison guard and as a community organizer. Whenever Sean is around on my visits to Sally's place, I find myself rather startled by his combination of grittiness, intelligence, curse words, and kindness.

Sally lives on her retirement pension and disability. She told me that she felt she was already in her ninth life, with her most recent near-death experience occurring only a few months earlier. At that time, her hemoglobin dropped precipitously and she was admitted to the hospital's ICU. When we met, she was just recovering from this medical crisis, but she has had many others, including a serious strep infection that had caused her entire body to go septic. This infection not only nearly killed her, but left her body paralyzed from the waist down.

After a long hospitalization, Sally lived for months in a nursing home in a small town near Lincoln. She had been isolated and wasn't receiving adequate care. She had been in so much pain that she could barely tolerate being covered by a shawl "woven out of spider webs." She had been sure she would die in that nursing home, but instead she was rescued by a nurse advocate who arranged for her to transfer to a hospital for better care.

Eventually Sally was able to return to Lincoln. Her friends helped her do the things she couldn't do for herself, and Sean, then in college, moved back home to care for her. He stayed with her for more than a year.

Before her health problems, Sally had lived a big life. She enjoyed international travel, had been married three times, and had many careers—running a restaurant, teaching, and writing. Over her lifetime, she has won literary awards and been a community activist. Recently she wrote the history of the Farmers Union of Nebraska. Now, one step at a time, Sally is reassembling her life. She consults with government officials about some of her professional specialties: agriculture, rural development, and global climate change.

Sally possesses the great gift of positive spin. Even her disabilities could be crafted into resplendent narratives. She said, "I enjoy the challenge of learning new ways to do things. It is a creative form of problem solving. As for my life, I have enough. I'll never be wealthy, but compared to the people all over the earth who live on two dollars a day, I'm a millionaire."

Sally was sixty-four and, when I asked if she saw herself as old, she said, "Yes. When I look in the mirror I see my grandmother. But it doesn't bother me because I loved her so much."

She told me she had acquired many survival tools. She was more empathic, but could also draw lines between herself and others for self-protection. As she put it, "I know the difference between you and me."

She was honest with herself. "I used to not know what to do with conflicting wants and needs, but now I have the ability to live within complexity," she explained.

"I am resilient. I don't panic when things go wrong," said Sally. She attributed this to her basic nature, but also to the twelve-step programs for adult children of alcoholics she participated in. Sally's mother was an alcoholic, and as an adult, Sally benefited from talking about the effects of her childhood.

Sally is not afraid of death. Having been near death many times, she knows that as death approaches most people feel too sick and miserable to be worried about dying. She believes what we all fear most is what she calls "psychic dismemberment," which is the loss of our identity, our ways of thinking, and our sense of self.

She recalled a dream she had as a nine-year-old. An aunt who had died of a stroke came to her in this dream and told her that people are not as afraid of death as they are of being forgotten. But, this aunt said, people are not forgotten. Rather their lives are like a flowered cloth that slowly fades. The pattern of their life remains on all the people they affected.

Sally helped her father through the dying process and made sure he felt as little pain as possible. A few minutes before his death, she and her stepsister were sitting beside him, talking about an old family friend. At the time, her father seemed comatose and they didn't think he could hear them. They were trying to remember the name of this old friend when her father said his name. He died peacefully right afterwards. Sally said that after that incident she always assumed that comatose people could hear and, in their presence, she made sure to be positive and loving.

Sally told me about one of her near-death experiences. She was embarrassed to tell the story because it sounded like something out of *Reader's Digest*. As Sally approached death, she saw light and the approaching shadows of people she knew who had died. When she was resuscitated, Sally was annoyed, because "Being almost dead was one of the most interesting experiences I ever had."

Still, Sally isn't sure what happens after we die. She believes we come from a great ocean and will return to it. We are connected to everything forever. Matter and energy are never lost. She laughed and said, "I am not sure whether we will be waves or particles but in some form or another we will go on."

Sally's idea of how she would like to be buried fits her quirky personality. As is the practice of certain Native peoples in our area, she would like a sky burial on the roof of her house so that the turkey vultures in her neighborhood can have a feast in her honor. But she and her son agreed that the neighbors might not like this. Her second choice was to simply be buried beside the tree in her backyard, but that's against the law. So she probably will be cremated.

The day of our interview, the sky was blue, the lilacs were blooming, and the grass was emerald green from a recent rain. Sally was feeling healthy at the moment. "Whenever I'm outside, I'm happy to be alive," Sally exclaimed. She mentioned seeing a small worm that morning on a plant and watching it quickly wriggle into the grass. She laughed, "It was in that worm's nature to be resilient, just like it is in mine."

Sally is almost too good to be true and most of us cannot rise to her empyrean heights of gratitude. However, I feel lucky to have met her. She still has a big life. Sally helped me put my problems in perspective. If Sally can be cheerful carrying the burden she does, then surely I can manage to be grateful and cheerful too.

Our True Heritage

Thich Nhat Hanh

The cosmos is filled with precious gems.
I want to offer a handful of them to you this morning.
Each moment you are alive is a gem,
shining through and containing earth and sky,
water and clouds.

It needs you to breathe gently
for the miracles to be displayed.
Suddenly you hear the birds singing,
the pines chanting,
see the flowers blooming,
the blue sky,
the white clouds,
the smile and the marvelous look
of your beloved.

You, the richest person on Earth,
who have been going around begging for a living,
stop being the destitute child.
Come back and claim your heritage.
We should enjoy our happiness
and offer it to everyone.
Cherish this very moment.
Let go of the stream of distress
and embrace life fully in your arms.

PART III

THE PEOPLE ON THE BOAT

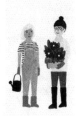

CHAPTER 14

Travel Companions

"I felt it shelter to speak to you." —Emily Dickinson

"Each friend represents a world in us, a world possibly not born until they arrive, and it is only by this meeting that a new world is born." —Anaïs Nin

For more than thirty years, Emma and her friends from the University of Colorado have camped in a state park to celebrate the summer solstice. They brought wine, Brie, and sourdough to their camping trips and, when the sky darkened, they built a big bonfire and sang around it. They slept in little tents under aspen branches and the stars.

During these trips, they told each other about the trials and victories of the year. They talked about their inner struggles, their spiritual beliefs, and their deepest reflections. This talking was a form of co-therapy. They educated, inspired, and healed each other.

Last year, Soledad told the group that she had been diagnosed with lupus and that her husband had terminal kidney cancer. The other women listened quietly as she explained the likely progression of her and her husband's diseases. Soledad was so upset she was shaking. Her voice kept cracking. Emma moved beside her and wrapped her arms around Soledad's shoulders.

When Soledad finished crying, Emma suggested the group hold a healing ceremony. Everyone but Soledad scattered along the lake to search for healing objects. A few minutes later, the women returned and gathered in a circle with Soledad. One by one they explained their gifts.

"This columbine stands for the beauty that will sustain you through anything," said Emma.

"This quartz is for the toughness that you'll need to endure the hard days ahead," said Lynette.

After the women offered their gifts, they looked into Soledad's eyes, placed their hands on her shoulders, and sent healing energy her way. Emma suggested that, with all of her troubles, Soledad needed a new name. She christened her "Courage."

This ceremony helped all of the friends. Soledad received healing gifts and a new name that would continue to give her strength. All of the women realized that this group would be there for them when it was their turn to have serious troubles. Emma thought to herself, "Only women our age possess the wisdom to design such ceremonies for each other. We could not have done this twenty years ago."

• • •

WOMEN HAVE ALWAYS worked together. For at least 200,000 years we have raised children, foraged for food, and walked for water with the women of our clan. As we rocked our babies, we sang together and, when our relatives died, we keened together. We talked at the edge of campfires and we listened to birds awaken at dawn. As we aged we helped with our grandchildren and watched the activities of our tribes' younger members.

We still love to be with our friends, but in the twenty-first century that requires planning and commitment. We often live far apart and have trouble finding the time to stay connected. Our culture doesn't teach us that our friendships are high priorities and that, especially as we age, they are what hold our lives in place.

But one by one, we discover the treasures of our female friends. With close friends, so many things need not be spoken. We can convey complicated, multilayered emotions with a look, an eye roll, or a smile. My friend jokes about how much conversation can be described as "talking and waiting for a chance to talk again." That doesn't apply to conversations with our gal pals.

I had close friends in junior high and high school, but I discovered my first soulmate in college. When I arrived at the University of Kansas the summer of 1965, I met my roommate, Janice. She was small, dark-haired, and dark-eyed, and vibrated with curiosity. She came from a blue-collar family in Kansas City and her father had not wanted her to go to college. She was the first girl I met who had read Tolstoy, Pasternak, and Dostoyevsky. She could recite poetry by Blake and Whitman.

Even though we were both shy in public, we were world-class talkers when we were alone. The first night in our dorm room we stayed up all night sharing our thoughts about life. After that eight-hour conversation, I realized that my life would be different. I understood that I was not the only person in the world like myself.

All of my adult life I have been nurtured by my women friends, many of whom I have been close to for decades. We go for walks, have long phone calls, and check in with each other daily. I can't imagine what I would do without them now.

Many of us found close friends in elementary school. We have our junior high besties, our high school and college confidants, and the friends we hang out with in our leisure time. Some of us are more introverted or have moved frequently and have only one or two close friends. However, no matter the number, it is when we reach our sixties and seventies that we most value our women friends. If we have children, they are grown; if we had careers, they are waning; however, if we are lucky, our friends are nearby and have time to see us. They help us keep things in perspective and even joke with us about our troubles. They freely offer us the companionship, understanding, and solace we all need.

In family relationships, we may be the caretakers and comforters, but our friends take care of us. The richness and joy of these relationships cannot be described in words. We can define wealth for women our age in terms of our time with close women friends.

No matter our age, we can select women who allow us to grow and to feel good in their presence. We can spend our time with women whose values we respect. I've always made the distinction between friends of the heart versus friends of the road—where circumstances have thrown us together. Friends of the road can be moms we met in a mother's group, colleagues at work, or someone on the same shift at the food bank. Of course, sometimes women who have been our friends of the road grow into our friends of the heart. On the other hand, soul-to-soul women can become close friends almost overnight. I know two women who met at a silent retreat. After this retreat, they walked toward each other, exchanged contact information, and agreed to plan a meeting. They have been dear friends ever since.

Friendship is really not a noun but a verb. Relationships of any kind require attention, energy, and time. If they are not nourished, they lose their value. When we are with our friends, we are always "friendshipping." That is, we are listening, sharing our own experiences, laughing, comforting each other, and enjoying the present moment. We are telling our friends we love and appreciate them. As I write this, I think of Louise who always brings her friends pastries the day they have biopsies or any other outpatient surgeries, or of my friend Gretchen, who signs off on her emails, "Thank you for loving me."

Women excel at troubles talk. We know how to listen and empathize. We can be each other's first responders in emergency mental health crises. We need not hide our pain, our flaws, and our unskillful behaviors. We can make mistakes without feeling that we are at grave risk.

Women friends help us define who we are. We end up sharing tastes in music, books, entertainment, and foods. We teach each other a continuing education course on how things work, and we motivate each other to dream big. With little gifts, compliments, and humor, we will encourage each other to take heart and carry on.

Friends remind us that there is nothing so terrible it can't be talked about on a walk or over a cup of coffee. As I write this, I think of the walks I had with my neighbor when my mother was dying slowly in a hospital three hours away. This situation made for a lot of stress and sorrow. But when I was home, after my family was settled in for the evening, Betty and I would go for a walk under the stars and I would tell her my tale of woe. She would listen sympathetically but also make jokes about my sorrows. At first, I found this shocking, but soon I eagerly awaited this chance to laugh. After those walks, I could sleep at night.

Carrie is an example of a woman whose friends pulled her through. She was sixty-four when her husband left her for a student from one of his classes. Throughout her troubled marriage, Carrie had suspected Bruce was having affairs, but they had never led to serious relationships. In spite of his dalliances, Carrie thought they had a good marriage. They'd raised three successful kids, enjoyed their seven grandkids together, shared a community of friends, and had a lively sex life.

A pretty woman with long black hair, Carrie had dressed fashionably and kept herself fit. But after one short conversation on a snowy morning, she was adrift. Her confidence and sense of invincibility disappeared. She quickly gained twenty pounds and drank red wine by the liter. She cried so much her eyes were permanently red around the edges.

Fortunately, Carrie's many women friends rallied around her and kept her from plunging over a waterfall of grief. One of them ate dinner with her every evening and they gathered for group coffees every Saturday morning. Carrie told them, "I'm going to give myself six months to feel angry, lonely, and afraid. Then I am moving into a new phase of life."

For those six months Carrie agonized over questions such as, "What did I do wrong? Why hadn't I seen this coming? How could I marry such a rat? Can I ever trust a man again?"

Carrie raged, cried, and indulged in revenge fantasies. She worried about her looks, her bank account, and her sanity. But she talked to friends daily, and in six months, just as she predicted, she was ready to move forward.

One evening, around dinnertime, she and Elise, her friend of twenty years, decided to plant a vegetable garden in Carrie's backyard. It was a fun project that had the two women working side-by-side most of the summer. Most evenings around dinner, Carrie sat on the front porch of the couple next door. She switched her beverage from red wine to sun tea. She started bicycling and lost her "trauma weight."

Carrie discovered that sunlight, warmth, and the color green were curatives for her. She felt her best when she was outside biking, porch sitting, or working in her garden. But then, cold weather came. The tomato vines withered, the bike trails iced up, and her neighbors stayed indoors.

Carrie rattled around in her three-bedroom house like a stone in a bucket. She pondered what could help her through the Pennsylvanian winter and realized it was her gal pals. She opened her house to her book club and a tai chi group. She refashioned a study into a meditation room and opened the library room to women who wanted to simply be alone to read or write. Indeed, Carrie's house became a women's retreat center.

Carrie relished her power to define her life in any way she wanted. She had never had this freedom before. She became a vegetarian and cooked exactly what she liked to eat. At night, she went to movies, concerts, and dinners. She was grateful she could afford to do this. She planned once-a-month slumber parties where she and her friends stayed up late watching Jane Austen movies.

However, she missed having someone around for coffee in the morning and a late-night chat by the fire. After careful consideration and multiple discussions, she invited Elise, who was also divorced, to move in with her. Carrie said, "We managed our conflicts over who did the weeding, so I figured we can handle any new tensions that crop up." She added softly, "I trust her."

After a year, Carrie felt happier than she had been when she was married. She was proud of her resilience in bouncing back and her creativity in designing a new life for herself.

Of course, Carrie and Elise had occasional disagreements, but the beauty of women's friendships is that we need not be perfect to stay with each other. In fact, success in long-term friendships requires that we accept others for who they are. If our expectations are too high, everyone disappoints us.

Old friendships can become rather habit-bound and dusty if we can't invent ways to experience change and growth together. We can invite new people into our circle. When this happens, group dynamics change and conversations become more exciting. Another good way to freshen up a friendship is to do something together we have never done before, such as visiting antiques stores or taking a road trip. Or we can bring up new topics of conversations, such as, "If you wrote history, what stories would you tell about the world?" or "What natural talent do you wish you could have developed?"

My friend Marge and I meet for lunch once a month and then visit an art exhibit. We look at the art together and share our reactions to it.

A surprising number of fresh topics and observations arise from these trips. We've known each other thirty years and it's fun to always have something new to discuss.

Women often are the connectors between neighbors of both sexes. I've met many of my best men friends through my women friends. Betty was the uber-connector in my neighborhood. She organized parties and made sure our neighborhood was a close and lively one.

Betty and her husband, Cal, hosted one last New Year's Eve party in their hundred-year-old stone house. They planned to move to a condo downtown in March. No doubt, they would host parties there too, but the parties would be different. We would be different.

When we moved into the neighborhood in 1980, Betty dropped by and invited me over. At that time, our mothers were alive, our hair was brown, and we liked to stay up past midnight. My son was nine and my daughter was three. Betty had young kids too and, over the years, we watched them all grow up, get married, and start families.

When we met, Betty was Election Commissioner. Later she directed our community action program and now she runs a nonprofit. I was a private practice therapist who had never written a book or given a speech.

Betty and I both smoked together and quit smoking together. We worked on human rights' campaigns and bought plants for our gardens. I was around for her kitchen remodel and she was around when I had my first book tour. We comforted each other during our many family crises. I attended Betty's seventieth birthday party when, as a joke, every single guest showed up with her favorite appetizer—artichoke dip.

It was dark and cold when I walked to Betty's house on that New Year's Eve. The pines, pummeled by the north wind, were stooped over like old men. But the house was lit up like a cruise ship and I could see pots of bright flowers though the windows.

Betty met me at the door in a sparkly red jacket. She was the least domestic person I had ever known and she regarded me as gifted and heroic because I could unwrap cheese and make guacamole. As I arranged things on plates for her, she carried them to the table in the wood-paneled dining room.

Cal walked into the kitchen to check on his roasting chickens. We shared our news of the day. That morning he'd had a biopsy for thyroid cancer and I'd called my doctor about blood pressure troubles. Then, we reminisced. Betty recalled that in 1973, after protesting with AIM and the Lakota at Wounded Knee, Marlon Brando came to a party in this house. He made himself a bologna sandwich and strategized about the events on the Pine Ridge Reservation.

As we talked, our old neighbor Bob stopped by with a cheesecake for the party. He had been a gregarious school psychologist, but now he is almost deaf. When I asked him how he was, Bob responded brightly, "Good." Then he paused and said ruefully, "Well, not really, but that is how it goes."

By eight, the front and back doorbells were ringing. Friends carrying food and wine rushed in from the cold night. Most of us met when we were in our vigorous thirties and forties. We were smart, energetic, and moving up. But now our energy was abating and we weren't moving up anymore. Our conversations were about health, vacations, retirement, and grandchildren.

Some of the neighbors had suffered great losses. Sue had lost her husband the year before. Other guests had cancer or disabilities or were struggling with Parkinson's or memory loss. No doubt a few were bitter about their lives or world in general, but they didn't speak of this at the party.

Instead we laughed and drank wine. We shared memories of past times and teased each other about our many peccadillos. We hugged each other and even sang "Auld Lang Syne."

I left the party just after that. As I walked home, I looked back on the ship of light. Through the frosted windows, I could see Betty's orchids, roses, and poinsettias and all my friends with their silver hair and bright sweaters.

The air smelled like snow. I knew a storm was coming during the night. It was the beginning of winter in Nebraska, but for now, I felt lucky. At the party, we shared what sociologist Émile Durkheim called "collective effervescence."

What makes me happy is what makes most people happy—a shared memory bank and people whose eyes light up when they see my face. Those people can be friends or family members. What's critical is the shelterbelt of loving relationships that are there for us when we need and want them.

CHAPTER 15

Co-Captains

"A long-term marriage has to move beyond chemistry to compatibility, to friendship, to companionship. It is certainly not that passion disappears, but that it is conjoined with other ways of love." —Madeleine L'Engle

"It's wonderful to be married to an archaeologist—the older you get the more interested he is in you." —Agatha Christie

EMMA WAS CHOPPING vegetables for a stir-fry when Chris came home from work one night looking tired and stressed. When she asked him about his day, he just groaned.

Chris started thumbing through the mail on the counter and found a Visa bill that showed that Emma had spent more than $100 on meals out with Alice and the twins. "I'm not made of money," he grumbled.

Although she was tempted to snap at him, Emma had been married for a long time. She knew this wasn't about the money, but about his day. She stopped chopping and walked over to him. She gave him a hand squeeze and said, "Oh, honey, I'm sorry you had a bad day."

Chris softened too and he patted her on the back. He managed to give her a weak smile and say, "Dinner looks good."

Later that evening as Chris dozed in his chair, Emma looked at him. When she met him, she was nineteen and he was a muscular black-haired college student. He could carry her around as if she were a snowflake. He'd wanted to be an engineer, but when she became pregnant, he dropped out of school to work in a small landscaping business. He helped her finish college and supported the family during their son's first year. Then, during Emma's first year of teaching, she became pregnant again.

She could still see in Chris the delighted father of young children and the harried, and often angry, dad of teenagers who were in all kinds of trouble. She remembered him the day their son graduated from the Colorado School of Mines. He'd been so proud, but also wistful that he'd never had that experience himself. And she could see him now, a man with gray hair and wrinkles around his eyes. He had knee and back trouble now, but he rarely complained.

When they were younger they had fought over almost everything. She blushed to remember the swearing and the raised voices. But now, they knew better. Both of them had become skilled at letting the little stuff go. They knew to cool down before they had a difficult conversation and, when they talked, they didn't interrupt or accuse. Even during an argument, they found ways to support and acknowledge each other.

Emma's work with her therapist on mindfulness helped her stay calm and, years earlier, marital therapy had helped them with communication. However, over the decades they had learned many lessons on their own. For example, they had learned to periodically simply ask each other, "Are you doing okay?" Then they would wait for a response and be prepared to listen as long as their mate wanted to talk.

Emma felt a rush of tenderness as she looked at the dozing and softly snoring old guy across the room with a cat on his lap. He was her old man.

• • •

SUCCESSFUL LONG-TERM MARRIAGES require women to skillfully navigate new relationships with our familiar, but evolving, partners. As life expectancy has increased, many of us are in marriages that have lasted forty or fifty years. Research tells us that the people who stay married are not those with the most perfect relationships, but rather, those who decide they are committed and stick with that decision. With this commitment and some skills, most marriages can be satisfying.

Marriages are the most successful when partners' interactions are mostly positive. Relationship experts John and Julie Gottman have documented the importance of this. They find that couples do best when they have ways to quickly emerge from negative interactions. Getting stuck in negativity creates a climate that fosters yet more negativity. On the other hand, being accommodating and complimentary is also self-perpetuating.

Neither trees nor people grow properly when they are planted too close to each other. Couples thrive when they give each other emotional and social space in which to grow. Not every decision needs to be mutual. A general guideline is that each partner is in charge of his or her own relatives when it comes to planning visits, buying gifts, or weighing in on major life decisions. Likewise, we all are in charge of our own bodies and free to choose our own friends.

Couple friends make marriages happier and more stable. Without family and outside friendships, marriages are forced to bear the entire weight of the emotional lives of the partners. Under those circumstances, the boat may sink. Yet, part of being attached to another person involves knowing when not to be attached. Time apart allows partners not only to pursue interests that may not be shared but also to have close friends.

Rita Rudner wrote, "I love being married. It is so great to find that one special person you want to annoy for the rest of your life." All marriages have conflict unless partners bury their disagreements and relate only in superficial ways. Simply understanding how to talk through a conflict keeps many a marriage alive and vibrant. Couples who have no tools to navigate conflicts often divorce from the simple buildup of ordinary frustrations.

Marriages last when couples are capable of honestly sharing their thoughts and feelings and of listening and empathizing without giving advice. During my years as a therapist, I remember thinking about how many marriages could be saved if both partners could just learn to say, "I hear what you just said."

Marriages in which partners know how to ask for what they want and need are more likely to be successful. Whenever I heard, "I want him to know what I feel without having to be told," I surmised that marriage was in trouble. We all need to be told by others what they want and need. We are not mind readers.

However, communicating well doesn't necessarily mean blurting out everything on our minds. One of the tricks for a happy marriage is not to say everything we are thinking. It never makes sense to be unkind or make gratuitous critical remarks. Likewise, it helps not to be easily offended by our partner's remarks. As Supreme Court Justice Ruth Bader Ginsburg said, "In every good marriage it helps sometimes to be a little deaf."

One of the great blessings of a long-term stable partnership is that people tend to balance each other out. The same personal traits that cause conflict also contribute to stability. In many couples, one person is the talker, the other the listener. Or, one is the emotional one while the other is low-key and nonreactive. This works as long as people don't get too stuck in these roles. The good talkers need to listen. The low-key person occasionally needs to demonstrate some deep feelings. Otherwise, our tendencies can lock us into rigid caricatures of ourselves.

People change. They grow, they learn, they develop new interests and opinions, and they often modify their expectations about relationships. At seventy, our partner is no longer the young, carefree person we met in college. Nor is he the beleaguered parent who can't find time to do the taxes or take us on a date. We aren't the same partners either. Many of us feel we have lived through multiple marriages, but to the same person.

Marriages can be difficult when one person is flourishing and the other is not. In these marriages, people can grow apart rather than together. In the best marriages, partners grow over the years and co-create each other. However, sometimes trauma stops that growth process for a while.

• • •

Sylvia and Lewis met in their church in Austin, married young, and grew up together. They had a good marriage for twenty years. After their daughter Lenore became a drug addict, Lewis and Sylvia suffered so much that they could hardly bear to be together; they saw deep reflections of their own pain in each other's faces. The weight of all that sorrow almost sank the marriage. Sylvia pondered divorce and Lewis became almost mute.

When their grandchildren came to live with them, Sylvia decided that she was not leaving. The children needed to be cared for and she and Lewis were the only ones who could do it. She would not have them in foster care. Raising their grandchildren was a goal that pulled Sylvia and Lewis back into a working relationship. They had strong Christian values; they loved the children and they wanted to raise them right.

Sylvia worked hard to stop nursing grievances. When she was angry with Lewis, she looked at a picture of him when he was a dimpled three-year-old smiling at the camera. That reminded her of his innate goodness.

Lewis helped the kids with their schoolwork and attended their swim meets. He played a little basketball with Max before dinner. That cheered Lewis up and helped Max settle down. Sometimes, as Lewis watched ball games or nature shows with the children, Gracie would crawl up in his lap and fall asleep.

One evening, after Max and Gracie were asleep, Sylvia went into the den to sit by Lewis. She asked him to turn off the TV and hold her hand. She said, "Lewis, we have so much to be grateful for. You are healthy and I'm becoming healthier. We don't have much money, but we are on Medicare and own the house. We can afford to keep the kids in swimsuits and tennis shoes."

Lewis listened carefully, then he started to cry. He said, "I've been so worried about you."

Sylvia handed him a Kleenex. She cried too as she said, "We raised Lenore the best we could and when she got in trouble, we tried to help her. She is not dead and may someday come home to us."

Sylvia awkwardly climbed onto his lap and embraced him. They held each other and wept. When they finished weeping, they kissed and stroked each other. Then, as Sylvia's knee jabbed Lewis in the stomach, he laughed and said, "We are like two old elephants trying to sit on a log." They broke into laughter.

On their forty-fifth wedding anniversary, Sylvia wrote in her journal, "Why did we do it? We were so different. Every decision has been a struggle. We've made each other miserable on a regular basis. Yet, it has not been all bad. We've had fun and good sex, and even though we frustrate each other, we still love each other.

"It is a tribute to our mutual affection that we are still together. In spite of all our problems, we have stayed, not out of habit, but because we wanted to be together. When we are apart, we miss each other.

"We have stuck it out. And not just for the grandchildren. Partly we are together because I'm afraid if I left Lewis, it would kill him. But if he left me, I'd have a terrible time too. We are two trees that have grown around each other.

"We have lived almost all of our lives and endured our most terrible moments together. Nobody but Lewis understands what my life is really like and I understand his life too. What else is there when we are old, except for someone who shares our history, joys, and sorrows, and who will be with us until the end?"

• • •

OUR TWENTY-FIRST-CENTURY MARRIAGES don't resemble those of our parents or grandparents. As the world has changed, so have gender roles and expectations about intimacy. Same-sex marriage is legal and divorce carries less stigma. And, in an era when we can earn our livings, women are partnered not by necessity but by choice.

In the last decades, psychologists' ideas about relationships have changed. In the 1980s, therapists encouraged couples to consider leaving relationships that were not fulfilling. They also encouraged partners to "let it all hang out" and share their anger and hurt feelings, no matter how trivial. Now our field has greatly tempered this philosophy. Today therapists teach the importance of reasonable expectations, ignoring the small stuff, and focusing on the positives.

Historian Stephanie Coontz maintains that "til death do us part" is a bigger challenge today. Divorce rates are declining for people in their prime child-rearing years but doubling for people over fifty and tripling for people over sixty-five. After the children leave, many people have thirty years of healthy life ahead and some realize they don't want to spend those years with their current partner.

Women initiate the majority of divorces and their most frequent complaints are their partners' lack of commitment or attention. Another complaint is that their mates are trying to exercise too much control over their lives.

Coontz concludes that the automatic advantages of getting married have declined and miserable marriages are a health risk. However, the advantages of a good marriage are increasing. When marriages are working, they improve women's health and wealth.

Barbara and Judy have been in a good relationship for thirty years, but only legally married since the federal government made same-sex marriage legal. Both of them are long-term Lincolnites embedded in a deeply supportive activist community.

In our conservative state, Barbara came out early as a lesbian. By her late thirties, she had tenure at the university and could afford to speak out. At that point, many gay men were dying of AIDS and she felt it was important to educate Nebraskans on gay and lesbian issues.

Meanwhile, Judy was married to a man and had a young daughter. Her women's group discussions opened her eyes to her true sexual orientation. After several months, she had the courage to come out. Soon after, she divorced her husband.

Barbara and Judy met in 1986 at a coming-out party, and in 1988, they had a wedding ceremony with all of their friends. When marriage became legal, neither Barbara nor Judy felt the need to acquire a marriage certificate, but they married in order to improve their tax situations and ensure medical power of attorney. They were the first same-sex couple to be lawfully married in our county.

Back in the 1980s, Judy's family had immediately embraced her relationship with Barbara, but when Barbara told her parents the news, her mother fainted. When she woke up, she told Barbara that the news would

192 Women Rowing North

kill her. That didn't happen, but her parents never acknowledged Judy nor allowed her to visit their home. In fact, the only time Barbara was able to speak about Judy was when she was at her mother's deathbed. Barbara said, "I sat by her side and told her what a wonderful person Judy was."

Barbara's experience with her own family motivated her to help other lesbians who were struggling with family and community prejudice. And finally, she and Judy formed a community of women who work together to advance good causes.

Now, Judy, who had polio at fifteen, uses a wheelchair. She can't go downstairs in their home or help much with household chores. Judy and Barbara no longer travel much. But they are both bird-watchers and they still go to nearby state parks for fall and spring migrations. They enjoy Judy's daughter, who lives in town. They host dinner parties for a community of women who have become part of their family.

They have been through a great deal together, including Judy's divorce, Barbara's family's ostracism of Judy, health problems, and discrimination. But their troubles have strengthened their commitment to each other. Their mutual respect, shared interests, and commitment to work on their marriage have kept their love alive.

• • •

My husband and I are also a long-term couple. We celebrated our fortieth wedding anniversary by taking a trip to the Pacific Northwest. We travel differently than many of our friends. We avoid cities and tourist areas and instead seek out the wildest, most remote places we can find. Once there, we spend our days hiking in silence, just looking at beauty.

On this trip, we made a point of sleeping beside water and we visited every old-growth forest or rain forest we passed. We stayed in lodges in Olympic National Park, then crossed over to Vancouver Island.

Our first two nights there, we luxuriated in a cabin at Kalaloch Campground in Olympic National Park. We were perched high on a cliff over a misty beach strewn with driftwood and shells. Just after we arrived I walked down to the beach alone. The area was empty—just me and the seagulls—but as I walked along the tide line, I noticed that someone had written the word "NOW" in big letters in the sand. Words from God on High couldn't have seemed more apt. NOW was exactly where I wanted to live for the next eleven days, not dwelling on the past or worrying about the future, but rather living in the senses, savoring the present moment.

That week we explored tide pools and found starfish, sea anemones, and hermit crabs. At night, we'd watch the sun set over the Pacific, then build a fire in our cabin's fireplace and listen to the ocean, which sounded ready to roll right through our open front door.

Mornings, we'd make sandwiches, fill our water bottles, and head out for an old-growth forest or rain forest. We walked for miles in dappled light, surrounded by silence and a hundred colors of green. We felt high on all the oxygen in those forests. Over time we learned to identify hemlock, ancient spruce, Douglas fir, and red cedar, a sacred tree to indigenous people.

At night, we dined in little cafés, often outside and sometimes by the water. One night at a café called Wolf-in-the-Fog in Tofino, I said to Jim, "We'll never be here again."

At the time, I meant that in the most prosaic sense. It was unlikely we'd ever be in this café in Tofino on a gorgeous September Saturday night. But later, I realized I felt a deeper meaning in that sentence.

We were in our mid-sixties and, at that moment, healthy and happy with each other and our lives. All of our close friends and family seemed healthy, too. Our children were in strong marriages and gainfully employed. Our grandchildren were loving and mostly well behaved. Just as that night in Tofino was golden, so was this larger September moment golden for us.

However, we were aging, along with most of our close friends, siblings, and cousins. When we got together with them we often talked of blood pressure, cholesterol, and checkups. In all likelihood, someone we loved soon would have a health crisis.

But that night in Tofino, the burdens of aging sat lightly on our shoulders. The benefits of life felt tremendous—time for the people we loved, time to read, and time to do the work we most wanted to do. This kind of wealth comes to children and to people who can slow down. Right then, Jim and I felt that richness.

Over the years, Jim and I have had our struggles. We have not had an easy marriage. I could not argue that we were meant for each other. However, that night we experienced a blessed moment in time. It was a good place to rest, made even better by the fact that we both knew the cold and darkness would come.

As I write this, I think of the foxes who live near us. They hunt together and share food. Every spring they raise a pack of kits together. Most important, on a winter night when it is blizzarding, they wrap around each other in their den and keep warm. Long-term couples are like foxes in a den who keep each other warm and safe.

Words cannot describe what it feels like over a lifetime to have someone to listen to us when we are troubled, protect us when we are down, and be with us when we face emergencies. This gift of security is as sacred and ineffable as moonlight. Sharon Salzberg wrote, "Real love is an ability, the capacity within us to deeply connect with another person."

CHAPTER 16

The Lifeboat of Family

"Call it a clan, call it a network, call it a tribe, call it a family.
Whatever you call it, whoever you are, you need one."
—Jane Howard

"Family life! The United Nations is child's play compared to the
tugs and splits and need to understand and forgive in
any family." —May Sarton

TOWARD THE END of what would be her last summer, Evelyn asked Kestrel to invite her brothers in California to come visit. Evelyn said she wanted to see all of her children together one last time. Kestrel hadn't seen her brothers in years, nor had she felt a deep desire to see them, but she called right away. When they quickly settled on a date, Kestrel was surprised by how grateful and relieved she felt.

That night, when Kestrel called Becca to tell her about the family reunion, Becca offered to drive from Seattle to help. Kestrel almost refused automatically. The thought of Becca being with her family for several days left her feeling claustrophobic and exposed. But Becca didn't give her time to protest. She rapidly moved into the topic of what she could bring—flowers, fresh salmon, and sourdough bread. Kestrel choked up at such tenderness. She said, "My mom loves Seattle sourdough."

The day before the family arrived, Evelyn went to the beauty parlor for a haircut and styling. Kestrel helped her pick out her prettiest comfortable clothes. Becca arrived and helped Kestrel prepare everything for the reunion. Kestrel was amazed by how good it felt to hug Becca's strong body and, for once in her life, to depend on another person.

In August Kestrel's brothers and their families burst out of their two big rental vans and into Evelyn's arms. Kestrel hugged everyone and so did Becca, who acted just like a family member. Kestrel had not seen her nieces and nephews in five years. Tim's oldest daughter had twin babies. Darren's youngest boy was starting high school.

Everyone was tired and hungry and Kestrel announced that dinner was ready. They were having salmon and lasagna. Becca chimed in that, with Evelyn's instructions, she had made chocolate pies, a favorite dessert in the family for sixty years.

During the visit, Evelyn's only assignment was to enjoy everybody. She held the twins on her lap in her big recliner or held her sons' hands as they talked. She played dominoes with the older grandchildren. Becca washed a lot of dishes while Kestrel talked to her sisters-in-law and nieces and nephews, who were growing into interesting people.

Family members occasionally left the room to compose themselves or cry, but when they were together, there was a lot of joking and laughing. One night, after a meatloaf dinner, Becca convinced the family to play a game of charades, but Kestrel was hesitant. She didn't believe that her family was "that kind of family" and she was mad when Becca pushed it. But she held her tongue and, to her surprise, her brothers agreed. Soon she joined the others in clowning around. She was surprised when Evelyn laughed at some of the rather sexual humor involved. They all laughed. When the game wound down, Kestrel realized that her family was much different, and much more fun, than the one she pictured from earlier years. Until this visit, she hadn't realized how much she had needed a family or how safe a good family could make her feel.

Three weeks after the family reunion, Evelyn fell into a deep sleep after a dose of morphine for pain. Kestrel lay down by her and held her hand. Evelyn died a few hours later.

Kestrel had a small ceremony for her mother at the mortuary chapel. Becca was by her side. The rest of the family didn't return for this. They had been with Evelyn when she was alive and could enjoy them. Instead they sent Kestrel a photo book of their happy times together.

• • •

KESTREL CAME LATE to an appreciation of family, but so do many of us. As we age, we tend to appreciate family more and to have more curiosity about family history. We sense that we are a link in a great chain and that understanding that chain helps us understand ourselves.

Family gives us our original source of identity. We belong to some people and they belong to us. We need not achieve anything to be part of this group. A "good enough" family gives us a shelterbelt, a circle of tall trees that protects us from the cold and wind. Over time, some of these trees die, and the tree line thins for a while. Then, we become the old trees. New trees pop up and grow to protect children who we may never meet.

Let's define family as the people we were raised with, are related to, or have adopted. Families can provide us with our deepest happiness and our greatest pain. Losing family hurts the most. Arguments and conflict with family stress us the most. Worries about family members' well-being can cost most of us many nights' sleep. And yet, when people are happy and enjoying each other, families provide one of the best experiences we can have.

Families are the people who will pay our rent if we can't pay or take us in after a surgery. They display our artwork or bowling trophies in their dens. They are proud of us when we complete a quilt or win a pie-baking contest. And they will be there if we call them from a hospital bed or during a dark night of the soul.

We do not need to like all of our family members. Who does? Especially as we get older, we can select the people who we want to consider as family. We may be connected to one sibling, but not to others. We may have family reunions with one side of the family, but barely see the other side. The important thing is that we have people who share a common history with us and upon whom we can depend. No matter what our families are like or how difficult people are to get along with, we can almost always find at least one person to love.

Even if we have no siblings or close relatives, we can find family members over the years. We can "adopt" our own brothers and sisters, or nieces and nephews, from the many people we know from work, our neighborhoods, our churches, or friendship groups. One woman I knew who had throat cancer had no family, but her book club members rallied to her bedside. They took turns driving her to doctors' appointments and treatments and, at the end, sitting with her at hospice. When she died, her book club members washed her body and prepared it for burial.

Many of us have adult children and, while our relationships with them are often complicated, they are also deeply rewarding. Especially as we age a sweetness enters into these relationships. Our sons finally have permission to unabashedly love us, something they couldn't do in high school or in their twenties. Our daughters often know us very well and can anticipate our needs. We have the pleasure of seeing our children develop into adults with their own lives and unique adult personalities.

We do not need to be politically attuned with our close family members to get along. Some of my favorite family members are politically my opposites. We have tacit agreements not to proselytize, talk politics, or in any other way offend each other when we are together. We sense deeper resonances than ideologies or common interests. We feel pleasure and comfort in just being together. My grandmother Glessie set the stage for this when she said, "We all belong to the political party of fried chicken and biscuits."

When my cousins and I get together for a reunion, we spend most of our time talking about our grandma and our parents. We savor long conversations about events that happened when we were together in our childhood. We look at old pictures and share family recipes. My cousin Steve cooks us the same big breakfasts my grandmother made us when we were kids.

When I am dispirited, I make my mother's vegetable beef soup. When I was growing up, she made it all through the winter. She prepared it with whatever ingredients were available but, at the same time, this soup always tasted like "my mother's soup." No one else could achieve her flavor. Now, in winter, I make vegetable beef soup with whatever I have around. I often add fresh mushrooms and kale, vegetables that weren't available to my mother in the 1950s. My soup tastes like hers and, when I serve it, I am with my mother.

Remembering those who loved us can be comforting. Or, if not comforting, it can be enlightening. We can feel grateful to those who helped us. We can try to understand those who hurt us and we can work to heal any broken relationships before it is too late. In this life stage, we are coming to terms with our whole life stories and we want them to be as rich and deep as possible.

Our most disastrous family stories explain a great deal. For example, one friend never understood her parents' hatred of alcohol until she found a yellowed newspaper clipping about her maternal grandfather. He had killed a man in a bar fight while he was drunk. For his crime, he was hanged in the courthouse square. Her mother had always told her that he died of Spanish flu.

When we are curious, we find multiple ways to explore the past. We can look into genealogy, have conversations with people who remember things we don't, or create experiences for ourselves that connect us to our past.

Most families have a family historian or three. In my family, it's my daughter-in-law, Jamie, my granddaughter Kate, and me. We are the ones who save the letters and old pictures and tell the family stories.

It's easy to become a family historian—just appoint yourself and get to work.

People come and go. If we are lucky, someone in our family has a Bible or other book that contains a list of the births and deaths of family members going far back in time. I started one for my family the year my mother died. I record everything in my *Webster's Third New International Dictionary*.

Letters are an excellent source of history. Many families have some around somewhere if only we dig. My mother saved all of my letters to her from the time I was seventeen on. She threw them in a barrel, and at the time of her death, I dumped them into a huge suitcase. When I read through them, I recovered a vision of myself through the decades. My father's sisters saved his letters from WWII, and I have a few war letters from my father to my mother. These letters give me a sense of my father's personality long before I knew him and also a window into a historical period of great significance.

Looking through old pictures can also unlock the past. Many of us have photo albums filled with black-and-white photos of stern-looking ancestors. As we examine these pictures, many questions come to mind. Mysteries may be untangled and secrets unearthed. For example, examining old photographs with my cousins, I found out that my dad had been married before he married my mother. No one told me that until I asked about the photo of him with a pretty dark-haired woman.

My parents both died before any of their siblings. When I was in my early fifties, I was able to interview all my aunts and uncles. I asked what my parents were like when they were young. What was their marriage like? What was I like as a baby and young girl? Did they remember any particular moments with my family?

As we age, many of us feel a need to keep our circle of kin strong and vital. Every year I host a reunion with my Ozark cousins. All are older than I am. All of them once changed my diapers and they have quite a lot to say about me as a little girl. They help me fill in memories about their families, our family history, and my family of sixty years ago.

We can visit sites that connect us to family history. I have returned to the small towns I grew up in and reconnected with old family friends. I have written letters to my mother's friends to ask what they remember about her. And, because I live in the state I grew up in, I still run into people who remember my parents. Many tell me that my mother was their doctor when they were young. I ask them what she was like as a doctor. People remember my dad as a philosopher, jokester, and opinion giver. They remember both his generosity and his anger.

Finally, we can build experiences that deepen our sense of family history. I've walked in Muir Woods where my parents were married in uniform. I've given speeches in Pearl Harbor, Tokyo, and Okinawa, where my father served. I've visited the graveyards and homesteads, the old houses, and the little stores, now mostly abandoned, where my relatives worked. When I can find a new place related to family, I explore it. Before we die, if we're lucky, we may be able to visit our ancestral homelands.

Garnet and Donald both grew up knowing their grandparents and they have close relationships with their local extended families. They also have worked hard through the years to make their marriage a deeply supportive one. And now, Garnet feels that they are harvesting the fruits of decades of parenting.

I visited this couple on a beautiful summer morning right after they retired—Garnet from teaching and Donald from surgical sales. Garnet smiled as she said, "When I wake up, I lie in bed and listen to the radio for a while. Then, when I drink my first cup of coffee, I ask myself, 'How can I enjoy my day?'"

Their cheerful demeanors and up-tempo conversations belie a traumatic past. Their son Jake was jumped and badly beaten while walking down a street in Chicago with his girlfriend. Their daughter Amy was injured and brain-damaged by the police while participating in a peaceful march in an East Coast city. It was many months before she could walk again. While Amy was hospitalized, one of them was always with her. They have worked together as a team to keep this family afloat.

Donald has been living with Parkinson's disease for seven years. He has a slight tremor and has slowed down some, but for the most part he still functions normally. He told me that Michael J. Fox was his role model. He's helping a friend who just received a Parkinson's diagnosis. He told her, "You can't control the disease, but don't let the disease control you."

Garnet had been the rock of the family, always strong for other family members. When tragedy struck, she had her trust in the universe and life skills at the ready. When the children were injured, she cried with Donald, but she said, "We'll get through this and be the better for it." When Donald was diagnosed with Parkinson's, she told him, "We're going to make this work."

If all I knew about this family were its factual history, I would think they were rather sad, but nothing could be further from the truth. No subject is unfit for comedy. One Christmas, the family laughed over watching the two children compete to prove who had been the most seriously injured. Jake had claimed he won because he had his medical records. Amy couldn't produce such a report on the spot. What a party!

Garnet was fascinated by her children's adult lives and, now that she was retired, she enjoyed more free time with family and friends. "I am embracing growing older," she said. "This stage is part of the circle of life. There are positives in every life stage."

"Where did you develop these master coping skills?" I asked them.

They laughed and shrugged as if to signal, "How the hell do we know?"

But they both talked about their childhoods and all of the family support nearby. They'd had many valiant role models. Donald's mother was a lifelong progressive activist. Garnet had grown up in a small town with a fun and loving family. Her brother had cerebral palsy; Garnet had been his advocate when he was young and his caretaker when he was older and lived in a facility in Lincoln. She and her brother dealt with his health situation by listening to music and having friends over. He was her shining example of flourishing through adversity. Loving a brother with health problems intensified her loyalty to family.

This couple had a quirky long-term plan for their family and friends. They wanted to buy a small town in Nebraska, not as far-fetched an idea as you might think since our state is full of empty little towns. In this town, they would all live together and take care of each other. Donald laughed and said, "And we could all take turns running businesses and governing the city. One week I'd be a cook, the next a banker, and the next mayor of the town."

While their plans for the future were sunny, they had their fears. Garnet had helped her mother through late-stage Alzheimer's and she was frightened at the thought of being unable to connect with the world in a meaningful way. Donald was already in physical therapy to mitigate the effects of his Parkinson's. "We all have to deal with what we are given.

I've seen many people adapt and be happy in their difficult circumstances," he said. "I'm not worried. Attitude trumps circumstance."

We talked about regrets. Garnet said she doesn't believe in them. "We
did things. Life happened but it doesn't make any sense to dwell on
regrets." She told a story about a time when Donald lost a job in Dallas
after his company went under. They lost their house and were stressed
by money problems, but she laughed and said, "At least our troubles got
us out of Dallas and back to Nebraska."

They relished their time with their son, who lives a few blocks away.
Donald and Garnet were helping him paint his house. He was a musician and he invited his friends over to play for his folks' parties. Many
nights a month they gathered with his friends and theirs to listen to
music, share food, and celebrate birthdays and retirements. "We never
feel alone," Garnet said, squeezing Donald's hand. "Friends and family
are everything."

Even when she discussed their sorrows, Garnet pointed out that these
have allowed their friends and family to show how much they love them.
They felt this most deeply when Amy was in an East Coast hospital after
her injuries. Everyone rallied to the family's side. They sent flowers
and chipped in frequent-flyer miles for the trips. When Amy finally was
able to come home, hundreds of people showed up at the train station
to welcome her.

Every year Donald and Garnet hosted a barbecue in their backyard
with live music. The invitation list topped 300 people. Just recently they
were invited to a party given by their son's friends and felt honored to be
the only older couple there. Donald said he believes in making friends
with every generation. That way as he ages he will never run out of friends
as his age-mates move or die.

"When we look at the children in our families, so much of what we
see is built of time," Garnet said. "We can see our relatives' features in
the bodies of the new children in our families. My cousin's three-year-old

reminds me of my brother at that age. My father's blue eyes shine in my grandnephew's face."

Our discussion ended with good news. Garnet told me that Amy was pregnant. We toasted this wonderful news with our lemonades. Donald said, "Now we'll receive the best gift life can bring, a local grandchild."

• • •

WHEN WE LOOK back, we can see generations of mothers and fathers who managed to take care of their children. We can see our ancestors working in peat fields, drumming around fires, fishing in faraway seas, or traveling by sled through fierce northern winters. We can see the Indian encampments of the Great Plains, the immigration or slave ships, and the grandparents walking west from the big East Coast cities.

We can say prayers of gratitude for our mothers and grandmothers and all of the mothers before them who gave us life. When we need strength, we can turn to them for inspiration and courage. We can remind ourselves that we come from strong stock. We wouldn't be alive today if we didn't.

We are adrift on a little boat rocked in the river of time, part of a long line of women who have lived in caves, swum in rivers, and foraged for food. We are the daughters of time, the children of mothers who fed us, rocked us, sang us songs, and kept us safe.

As we approach the end of our time, we can feel safe under the sky full of our ancestors. And some of us are becoming the ancestors for new generations of family.

CHAPTER 17

Grandchildren

"Heirlooms we don't have in our family. But stories we've got."
—Rose Chernin

"You can never really live anyone else's life, not even your
child's. The influence you exert is through your own life, and
what you've become yourself." —Eleanor Roosevelt

IN AUSTIN, SYLVIA continued to journal, swim, and meet with her women's
group on Sunday mornings. Even though she had significantly less pain,
Sylvia saw Megan, her pain therapist, every few months. She liked talking
to her and needed that prescription for the therapeutic swimming pool.
Every night she gave Lewis a short report on her physical pain and every
night he listened carefully, then sweetly acknowledged what she had said.

As her mental and physical health improved, she became more
grateful for her custodial grandchildren. Too often in the past, she had
allowed herself to think of them as a burden when, in fact, they were the
best thing in her life.

Gracie liked art and animals and she made friends easily. Max was
a tall, skinny kid with big ears and an awkward gait. He reminded Sylvia

of a baby giraffe—gangly, well-meaning, but unintentionally destructive. When he first came to live with Lewis and Sylvia, he had a dozen meltdowns a day, but now he only had one every few days. He was a restless, moody boy, but also warmhearted and funny. Sylvia took pride in how much better Max was now.

While she did her chores, Gracie sang tunes from *Annie* and *Mary Poppins*. She was full of life, a beam of sunshine that Sylvia could bask in whenever she wanted. Max read her jokes from his corny joke books while she cooked. One night, she heard him singing to himself while he played with Legos in his bedroom. That night she felt that she was a lucky woman.

• • •

OF COURSE, NOT everyone who has grandchildren is lucky. One of my friends is estranged from her daughter and is no longer able to see her grandchildren. She is so lonely that she has adopted three cats and named them after her two granddaughters and grandson. Another friend loves her grandchild, but he lives in Hong Kong and she has seen him twice since he was born five years ago. Some grandchildren are so badly behaved that it's painful to be with them. When adult children are not parenting well because of drug or alcohol abuse, criminal behavior, or mental health problems, grandmothers can feel despair. But these are the exceptions. Most of us are delighted by our grandchildren. They make us happier than we ever realized we could be.

I remember a story about Queen Marie Antoinette, who possessed an enormous collection of rubies and diamonds. One day a visitor asked to see her jewels. She had a servant bring in her children and said, "These are my jewels." That is how I feel about my grandchildren.

If we are lucky, our grandchildren light up when they see us. At least when they are young, we may be their favorite people. Unlike their parents, we don't have to be responsible for their daily lives. We can love them and they can love us back. At best, this relationship is one of the purest and most golden relationships possible. It has a sacred quality. We have special names for each other and many of our activities become ritualized.

Part of what sanctifies these relationships is that we have learned to let our grandchildren be perfectly themselves. We may have tried to shape and form our own children into mini-versions of ourselves, but by now, we know better. Instead, we accept our grandchildren for the unique beings they are. This acceptance gives them the confidence to feel they are worthy of the deep love they are given. It helps them see the universe as safe. It is the psychological equivalent of being given milk and cookies before bed and tucked in with a story and a kiss. This core confidence and sense of self-worth stay with children for the rest of their lives.

If we are fortunate, we remember our own grandmothers with whom we had special relationships. As a grandmother now, I am realizing how much my grandmothers loved me. The good things that happened when I was with them were not accidents. Rather, when I was there, my grandmother would decide she wanted to make gooseberry pie. Then she and I could sit under her ash tree and de-stem the gooseberries while we visited. Later we could enjoy the delicious pie together.

The picnics and the trips to the river with my Ozark grandmother required work and planning on her part. She was intentional when she asked me to talk to her while she weeded her garden or ironed other people's clothes in her dark kitchen. As a grandmother now, I know how much work it takes to make events for children "just happen."

My grandmothers bequeathed me memories around specific activities, places, and conversations. I treasure these memories. I've passed on to my own grandchildren some of their songs, stories, and card games. As I grew older, both grandmothers asked me questions about myself, such as how did I choose my friends, what did I feel passionate about, what books I enjoyed and why, and what did I think my talents were? I grew after these questions. I have tried to ask my own grandchildren questions of a similar caliber.

We grandmothers can ponder what it is we most want to teach our grandchildren, what activities will give them the most joy, and in what ways can we prepare them for life in our complicated world. As we think through these big questions, we will be able to, day by day, share with our grandchildren what we most want them to experience.

We can offer our grandchildren the gift of slow time, something schools and busy parents are not always able to do. We can allow children to live in the present with uninterrupted attention from us. Children appreciate unscheduled time and the opportunity to complete tasks without being interrupted.

We can also help parents keep things in perspective. We can remind them that they were fidgety at the dinner table, too, and hard to get to bed at night when they were toddlers. And we can reassure them that as parents we made many mistakes and yet they managed to survive our parental imperfections to become the wonderful people they are today.

We can invent new rituals. When I am with my grandchildren, we take nature walks with our water bottles, bird books, and paper bags for carrying the treasures we find. We pick up colorful stones, acorns, and leaves. When the children go on vacations they bring back these kinds of treasures to me. In the summer, we deadhead the red and pink hibiscus and have flower fights with the soft fallen flowers. In the autumn, when ginkgo leaves turn golden, I gather a few and mail them to the children.

My grandchildren have their favorite foods that I keep handy for them. For my son's children, it is bagels, yogurt, and oranges. My daughter's children like pitas, Goldfish crackers, and applesauce. I do not run out of these foods. They are sacramental.

Glenda and Doug are retired grandparents who live five blocks from their grandchildren. Like many boomer grandparents, they are deeply engaged with their grandchildren. Last summer, when the grandchildren were too old for daycare, Glenda and Doug offered to watch them. They planned a summer of exploration. They wanted the children to see new places, experience new activities, and learn about their city.

They picked up the kids around nine a.m. with a plan for the day. They took them to museums, bookstores, and free concerts in the park. They drove to a climbing wall, a zip line course, and a weekly karate class. Glenda wasn't fond of martial arts, but the kids loved it.

As they drove around their city, Glenda and Doug would point to things the children might not notice on their own. One day they looked at streetcar tracks and talked to the children about why streetcars were such a good idea. Another day they took the children to the farmers market and encouraged them to choose one vegetable they didn't think they would like. Glenda cooked it for lunch and let them see if they were right. After each day's activities, they all wrote about their experiences.

And the children give back to them. One day their granddaughter said, "I want to live with you when I go to college. I'll take care of you then." Another day, their grandson looked at Glenda and said, "Grandmother, you have a lot of wrinkles." Glenda replied, "I know. I am getting old." Then her grandson said, "I call them 'wrinkles of love.'"

We can offer our grandchildren a moral education, deepen their sense of connection to all living things, and help them learn to find comfort in reading, people, the natural world, and creative works. One of the best ways to do this is simply talking through questions about life. One day Coltrane asked me, "Do you believe God created the world?" and I responded, "I don't know." Then he said, "Maybe little specks came together and created it." Again I said, "I don't know." He asked me, "But who created the specks?" "My question exactly," I replied. We then talked for fifteen more minutes about the nature of believing, the existence of spiritual life, and our lack of certainty about both God and the creation of the universe.

Plato taught, "Education is teaching children to find pleasure in the right things." Grandmothers can be teachers about how to lead an ethical life. Partly we can do this by modeling kind and respectful behavior toward all living beings. We can also do this by storytelling. For all of my grandchildren I created a long and endlessly useful story about the Lovelies and the McGarigles. The Lovelies are a well-behaved family who are kind and sensible and know how to act in public. On the other hand, the McGarigles are rude, messy, lazy, and mean to each other. Before any new event such as attending a wedding, going to a new museum, or having a birthday party, I tell the children both versions of how the event goes. They find the McGarigles, who throw around their food and scream at their parents and sometimes belch and swear in public, to be hilarious. And they all promise they will act like the Lovelies at whatever event is coming next. Whenever I want those kids to behave, all I have to say is, "Act like a Lovely."

Another way to teach moral behavior is to tell what I call crucible stories about how people act when their backs are to the wall. Children love stories about orphans or any children who are brave and self-sufficient in difficult situations. I tell my grandchildren stories of adults who behaved well on the *Titanic* or an expedition to the South Pole or in modern disasters such as the Chilean mining accident where the miners took care of each other for many days before their rescue.

We also play a game called What If? I ask the children questions and allow them to tell me how they would behave in a challenging situation. For example, "What would you do if you were about to get in a car with an adult, but you realized she had been drinking?" "What would you do if you found $1,000 sitting on the sidewalk?" or "What action would you take if you woke in the night and smelled smoke in your house?"

Children love these games because they give them a chance to work out complicated and practical problems. This gives them more confidence in facing their future and prepares them for the events that might occur.

I favor conversations about how to protect a child who is being bullied, how to lose gracefully at games, and how to help people in need without offending them. My oldest grandchildren and I have discussed what to do if someone says something hateful or racist. We have discussed war as a terrible and often avoidable way to solve conflicts. We have talked about what it means to be a citizen.

Children have lives just as complicated as adults and face many of the same existential quandaries. Most are capable of empathy, reflection, and action for the good. Grandmothers can teach children to work by loving work themselves. Both of my grandmothers worked all the time, but while they worked, they had lovely lives of visiting and laughing. That is the kind of life I want to show my grandchildren. I talk to them enthusiastically about my writing and my volunteer projects and, when the children are here, I often suggest we work together. When we work with them, children love to work.

Grandmothers give children the great safety net of an inborn identity, woven of time, place, and people. One of our most important jobs is to talk to children about the six generations of family that we may know. The more storied a child's life is, the stronger and deeper are his or her possibilities for a rich sense of self.

We can teach our grandchildren the family value systems that span generations. All families worship at some church, be it a literal church, synagogue, temple, or mosque or the church of sports, music, fly-fishing, or good works. I watched my Colorado grandmother work as a volunteer at her church and library. I observed my own mother's constant generosity with others. When she left the house every morning for work, she would say, "Be kind to each other."

Far back in time, our family held certain values. We believed in hard work and kindness. We valued education, good food, and being outdoors. We treasured experiences over objects. We loved birds and we gathered to observe big storms and express wonder as the lightning crackled and the thunder boomed. I hope my grandchildren learn our values by watching me.

One night our tornado sirens twice interrupted our Mother's Day dinner. We raced to the basement. Four-year-old Coltrane had never experienced our trips to the basement with cats, flashlights, and cell phones. He'd never seen a meteorologist live on TV showing maps and red zones and warning people to seek shelter.

I was grateful to be with Coltrane on his first tornado night. That gave me a chance to educate him about our family's love of big storms. After the storm moved east of us, we walked around outside looking at the clouds. We marveled at the wind and the temperature drops. I said, "Storms are when nature shows us all it can do."

Children love to hear what their parents did when they were young and especially how they misbehaved. They like to hear about themselves— stories about their births, their early words, and their funny habits.

We are all cultural historians for our grandchildren. We remember the Mickey Mouse Club, drive-in theaters, John F. Kennedy's election, the Bay of Pigs, the Vietnam War, the Democratic convention of 1968, the Black Panthers, and the popularization of granola, yogurt, and, of course, kale.

We can tell them about the much slower and quieter world we lived in. My grandchildren can hardly believe my parents let me ride my bike down to a creek with only a book, a can of soda pop, and a peanut butter sandwich. I would spend the day reading under a tree. They are surprised to know that many houses didn't have locks on the doors and that people left their keys in their cars overnight.

I have told them about ten-acre prairie dog villages, bookmobiles, and teachers having to resign when they were pregnant. I have explained that girls had to wear skirts to school even on the coldest days of winter and that severely disabled children stayed home from school. And I have taught them the games from my rural childhood—Red Rover; Run, Sheep, Run; Statues; jacks; hopscotch; and tiddlywinks.

My grandchildren can barely comprehend a world without television, microwave ovens, power windows in cars, cell phones, computers, and air-conditioning. That is the world I grew up in. To them, my history is ancient history.

Our stories help children develop identity, perspective, and a point of view that will shape the way they understand their experiences for the rest of their lives.

Of course, grandchildren bring us as many gifts as we carry to them. Being around grandchildren rekindles our love for children, and reminds us of our own and our children's childhoods. Children also tend to bring a great deal of sheer goofiness into our lives. No matter how rough a day my husband and I have had, we can change the topic and cheer up by starting to talk about something funny one of our grandchildren said or did.

Grandchildren combat loneliness, make us feel young again, and give us a mission. In my own experience, there's nothing like a newborn baby. I love the pleasure of rocking an infant and feeling his or her head on my shoulder close to my neck. I enjoy the sound of babies breathing and, even though it means a bad night's sleep, I love to sleep with a baby curled beside me. And I will never forget the joy of walking around a garden with Kate in my arms.

No one but one-year-old Otis enjoys my singing and dancing to show tunes from the 1950s and 1960s—"Oh, What a Beautiful Mornin'," "I'm Gonna Wash That Man Right Outa My Hair," and "76 Trombones."

Babies have a lot to teach us—to love the people we love radiantly, be direct about our needs, and that the time to enjoy life is NOW.

Who is more fun than a three-year-old? At that age, Coltrane spent the night and woke me at five a.m. It was still dark and I seized the opportunity to take him stargazing in my front yard. We spread out a blanket and looked at the universe. Both of us were awestruck by the silvery moon, the many constellations visible in the pre-dawn sky and, well, by the bigness of it all. Later, I fixed cinnamon toast and we watched the sunrise. I hope to remember this on my deathbed.

At five, Coltrane discovered air quotes. We had a hilarious afternoon in which anything we said was in air quotes. It is astonishing how funny most ordinary sentences can be if they are air-quoted. Even the sentence "I want a snack" can be hilarious with the word "snack" in air quotes.

Ten-year-old girls are marvelous. When my granddaughter Claire was ten, she came in to visit for a week of art camp and swimming. One sunny afternoon, just before she dived into the pool, she gave me a hug and said, "I am the luckiest girl alive." I realized at that moment that I was the luckiest nonna alive to be with such a joy-filled and grateful granddaughter.

When my grandson Aidan was in middle school, he sustained a concussion. He was on a strict regimen for two weeks—no television, no school, no friends, and not much moving around. I called him every day and sent him packs of licorice in the mail. But finally, I just needed to go see him.

I drove ninety miles to his farm. When Aidan saw me, he walked toward me surrounded by a golden light. I could feel my heart open and my love for him beam out into his heart and beyond. We were so grateful to see each other and to hug. We needed to be together that day.

Aidan suggested we go fishing, one of the few activities he was allowed to do. I drove him to a little farm pond nearby and watched as he casted for fish. I spotted fish for him and admired his skills. But truly, all that mattered for either of us was just being together. I will remember all of my life that afternoon with Aidan fishing in the sunlight filtered through the light green leaves of spring.

Teenagers are fun too, although we grandparents stop being the center of their universe. Friends and activities replace us. It's hard to let go of the physically affectionate, crazy-about-me grandchildren that my teenage grandchildren once were. A part of me wants to hold on to the loving and deeply connected children of the past.

However, I have worked to adapt to their changes. I've told them that I want them to be honest and authentic with me. I want to know what they really feel and think. I don't want the edited version of their lives. I feel closer to them when I hear of their struggles. That is the only way we can stay truly connected as people.

I am working to find new ways of being with them. I don't want to just love the memories of my young grandchildren. I want to love and understand the people my grandchildren are becoming. I stay engaged by going to their sports events and by learning about what they are interested in. Kate and I sometimes read the same book at the same time so that we can discuss it. Aidan and I like board games. When the family visits, I try to find half an hour to be alone with each of the teenagers. My husband and I also have a custom of taking each of our grandchildren on a trip when they are in high school.

Grandmothering requires constant adjustment. Children change and so do we. I am not the same grandmother for toddler Otis that I was for Kate, my oldest grandchild. When Kate was a baby I was fifty-four; now I am seventy.

As the children have changed, I have worked to keep my expectations reasonable, not too high or too low. For example, at age three, children are old enough to help set and clear the table and they should be contributing to family work. On the other hand, I know that children don't always enjoy what I hope they will enjoy. When we took our thirteen-year-old grandson to an old-growth forest, he loved to find and hold banana slugs. By the time our hike was over, he had counted seventy-five banana slugs and been photographed with many of them. I might have focused on the lovely moss backlit by sunlight or the redwood branches swaying gently in the wind, but he was a young kid and slugs were more exciting.

Even in the best situations, grandmothering is complicated. My multigenerational family can make me happier and drive me crazier than anything else on earth. I look forward to family gatherings and often have a glossy fantasy about how they will be. At the same time I am fearful because historically family gatherings are sometimes fraught with hard moments. High expectations can cause me trouble. Unless I control that, I can end up weeping after a big family holiday.

Grandmothering requires great diplomatic skills and self-discipline. We learn to be quiet. We learn that our main talking points need to be "You have wonderful children" or "You are great parents."

My friend Regina plans to have her grandchildren call her Grandma Chocolate-money. My friend Jane recommends keeping your criticism to yourself, but being generous when it comes to picking up the tab at the ice-cream shop or paying for special learning opportunities for the grandchildren.

Roles have switched and now our children are the authorities. We do as they wish with the grandchildren and we don't question their authority. Unless asked, we don't offer advice. As my Buddhist friend said, "My mantra is 'I am not being called upon to issue an opinion.'"

Somehow, we must learn to balance our great love and concern for our grandchildren with the acceptance that we are not in charge. We control almost nothing. Especially when we feel like we know something that could be helpful, it's hard not to share our thoughts. But, as my daughter once told me, "Mom, none of my friends want their mother's advice on parenting unless they ask for it."

We can be most helpful when we are praising, chauffeuring, preparing food, introducing children to cultural events, and supporting tired and stressed parents.

Children who are loved and well-parented can survive a considerable number of parental errors in judgment. It helps to remind ourselves that we don't know everything and that our opinions are not always correct. We can remember the many mistakes we made as mothers. We wish we could save our children from trial and error learning, but we cannot.

Our grandchildren grow up so quickly. With each developmental leap they make, we lose the child we were in love with. We lose the three-year-old who likes to sit on our lap and read library books or the eight-year-old who is endlessly performing magic tricks. Those children disappear and new ones appear. I am already through the baby stage of my life. Unless I live to be very old, I will never have another grandbaby to rock.

When my husband and I were the parents of younger children, we often commented on how much our parents wanted to see us. They were always urging us to visit, and when we arrived they would be standing on the porch or looking out the window, waiting for our car. When we left, they would walk us to our car and talk as we fastened our seat belts. We had a hard time extricating ourselves and driving away. Now I am like my parents, watching out the window and crying when the family leaves.

PART IV

THE NORTHERN LIGHTS

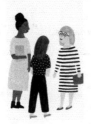

CHAPTER 18

Moon River: Authenticity and Self-Acceptance

"I think that somehow, we learn who we really are and then live with that decision." —Eleanor Roosevelt

"I am luminous with age." —Meridel Le Sueur

ONE MORNING, AFTER a hike in the Rockies, Alice asked Emma to buy her a gym membership so that she could work out. While that seemed like a reasonable request, Emma had a long history of buying Alice memberships to zoos, aquariums, and recreation centers. Alice would go a few times and then lose interest.

Emma frowned and Alice said, "Mom, this time I'll stick with it."

Emma's natural impulse was to give in, but, after a year of therapy, she was more grounded. She acted on the basis of reason, not fear of disapproval. She told Alice, "You pay for the first couple of months and then, if you are using the gym regularly, I'll pay half."

Alice looked surprised by Emma's response, but she didn't protest. Instead she said, "I'll think about it."

Emma felt a burst of pride. She had listened to her inner voice and set a reasonable limit with her daughter. "Pat yourself on the back, Emma," she said to herself.

As Emma became more honest with herself and others, Chris responded in ways Emma wouldn't have predicted. He was pleased that she was taking better care of herself. He said, "You're more fun when you're not stressed all the time. I'm not as worried about you."

Alice respected her more and stopped being so snippy. It seemed to Emma that Alice had been testing her to see how far Emma would go before she pushed back. Now that Emma had established boundaries, Alice didn't need to test. She asked Emma for less and was more grateful for what Emma did offer.

Emma's yoga, massage, meditation, and journaling have helped her stay in touch with herself. At last, in her seventh decade, she is learning who she truly is.

• • •

ONE OF THE great gifts of our later years is the possibility of authenticity, or what Margaret Fuller called the "radiant sovereign self," which comes from growing out of fears into wholeness. We may lose our false selves, acquired in childhood and carried with us through much of our long journey. We have the potential to discover our true selves deep inside and, at last, be able to tell the truth.

By engaging in the process of becoming more integrated and aware, we learn that the most important relationship is the one we have with ourselves. At the same time, paradoxically, we are likely to lose our youthful narcissism and self-involvement. We process and integrate our own experiences into a deeper sense of both who we are and what the world is. We gain skills in regulating our own emotions and setting healthy boundaries between ourselves and others.

As in all developmental challenges, growth requires both an existential choice and a set of skills. No matter what happens to us, we can all make the choice to grow. When we stop worrying so much about what other people think, we grant ourselves permission to live just as we truly are. We can acknowledge and accept our negative emotions and flaws, but also our deep desires to be honest, joyful, and free.

Finally, we can give ourselves permission to spend time with only those people we truly enjoy. We can chortle with our friends, buy ourselves flowers, and dance to the music of the moon. By paying attention to our ordinary surroundings, we can find splendor in daily events.

Authenticity means different things to different women. To Maria, it means not dyeing her hair, dressing up, or attending events she doesn't want to attend. To Yetta, it means sleeping in on Sunday mornings and eating pie for breakfast if she feels like it. When Naomi finally stood up to her bullying husband and informed him she'll move out if he doesn't quit, she felt whole and free. Jill feels authentic when, without an apology, she shares her pain and anxiety with others.

For frosty Kestrel, authenticity meant learning to trust. Until the summer her mother had cancer, Kestrel had only trusted herself. She had been comfortable with her anger, but she couldn't stand vulnerability or tenderness. She had inhabited a small fortress of self, surrounded by a moat filled with red wine.

However, Evelyn's cancer cracked open the gates to Kestrel's locked heart. In caring for her mother, Kestrel healed herself. She became whole, a person who could trust and who could be vulnerable.

At first, her new tender emotions were frightening. If she had known how, Kestrel would have relocked the doors to her heart. But this time she couldn't ignore her own sorrow. What had started as worry about her mother expanded into a portal into her complicated, emotional, and vital self.

• • •

FOR SAL, AUTHENTICITY was finding the God she had sought as a child. When I met her in New York City, she was dressed in black slacks and a tangerine-colored jacket. Sal had a kind, sincere face and she thought carefully before she answered questions. She could be witty but, for the most part, she was earnest and intense. The first thing Sal said was, "I should have been born a six-foot, four-inch-tall guy, but instead I was born a short woman."

She believed the disconnect between how she saw herself and how she looked had caused problems throughout her life. She felt she had internalized some of the culture's views on short people. Being so small, she felt diminutive. She was aware that the word "short" was sometimes used as a synonym for "lacking," as in short-changed or short-circuited.

She resisted cultural pressures to be feminine. As a girl, she refused to wear dresses or have her hair curled. She wouldn't play with dolls. "That wasn't me," she told me. Now she dressed more like a man than a woman and kept her hair cut short.

As a child, Sal was sexually abused by an uncle for many years. She told her mother about this abuse three times, but her mother did not believe her. The fourth time she brought it up her mother slapped her and told her to stop telling lies.

The week after high school graduation Sal moved to New York City. She lived on the streets until she was offered a job cleaning in a busy salon. She allowed herself to be exploited sexually. She suffered such a low opinion of herself that she felt she deserved to be treated like a sex object.

She possessed no understanding of personal boundaries and was afraid of being close to anyone. She was not connected to anyone.

Sal said she had blocked out a great deal of her past. She remembered almost nothing about her middle school years. "When I look back on my life, I see darkness and pain," Sal told me. "I was an outsider. I was assaulted, insulted, and bullied. I am amazed I am here today."

What held her life together was her Catholic faith. As a girl, she wanted to be a priest. She said Mass in her living room and practiced the various prayers that priests used. Praying and enacting rituals of the church comforted her.

By the time Sal was ten, she knew she was a lesbian, but she kept quiet and hid her feelings toward other girls. When she was twenty-four, she married and tried to be straight. In the 1970s, she gave that up. She came out at a time when being a lesbian in New York City was about bars, drugs, and the counterculture. She wasn't prepared for that and quickly became an alcoholic.

Through the '80s she was a hairstylist for gay men in the city. She had many famous clients from Broadway and the arts community. In that decade of AIDS, 70 percent of her clients died. She lost her friends and her business was wiped out. Now that she is in her sixties, many of her friends are worried about losing friends and her response is "That's already happened to me."

Thirty-three years ago, Sal went through alcohol treatment and joined an AA group. Now Sal leads twelve-step workshops and organizes groups for women who have been sexually assaulted.

Her successful relationships began with AA friendships. When she attended the seventieth anniversary of AA in Toronto, she met an outgoing dynamo named Norma, who was fourteen years younger than she. The last night of the convention they talked all night long. The next morning, they departed for their separate cities but they continued their relationship through phone calls to each other. A year later, Norma moved to New York City to be with Sal. Norma is Sal's first and only long-term partner.

The last ten years Norma and Sal have lived with and cared for Sal's mother, who has severe arthritis and is almost blind. Sal and Norma help her bathe, cook for her, and keep her company. Her mother is frail and loving; Sal no longer feels angry about her mother's lack of protection for her when she was a vulnerable child. Her mother is the vulnerable one now.

Sal has had serious health problems, including Epstein-Barr virus. She jokes that during her thirties she was "allergic to everything and could only eat twigs." Then she developed breast cancer and was forced to confront the fact that she might die. But slowly, with not only traditional treatment but also yoga and a macrobiotic diet, she returned to good health.

After Sal recovered from cancer, she knew how desperately she needed a connection with God and became a seminarian. Once she got her degree in ministry, she formed her own church. Once again, saying prayers and enacting rituals became part of her daily schedule.

On Sundays, Sal gives a sermon to her congregation. She also presides over wedding ceremonies, memorial services, and house blessings. She leads retreats and spends most of her time helping people with their spiritual growth. Her message is simply that we are worthy of love and respect.

Sal has grown much kinder to herself. She treats herself in small ways. For example, she's been taking pottery lessons and going out for sushi once a week. After all she has been through, Sal feels lucky to be alive. When she looks back on her earlier years, she realizes that she was looking for God in her alcoholism. "I have looked for God all of my life and now God blesses me with her presence," she told me.

• • •

No MATTER OUR circumstances, if we keep a green growing edge, we can make our lives complete and beautiful. Authentic lives result from a deepening process that requires us to listen to our bodies, our hearts, and our minds. One of the best methods for doing this is meditation, but any vehicle for self-awareness, such as artwork, journaling, yoga, or reflective conversations, will move us toward understanding who we truly are.

Self-awareness allows us to separate our own needs and desires from those of others. We can ask over and over again, "What part of this inter-action is about me? What part of this situation is not about me?"

These questions teach us to not take everything personally, and yet to also assume responsibility for ourselves.

We can learn the importance of checking in on ourselves on a contin-uous basis and to monitor ourselves for our own quirks, blind spots, and recurring stories. We can train ourselves to recognize our impulses and our destructive thoughts without feeling a compulsion to act upon them. We can be aware of our judgmental nature, yet stop ourselves from actu-ally judging. We can pay attention to that voice deep inside us that wants to protect us and take good care of us.

By the time we are sixty-five, we are likely to know how to enjoy ordi-nary days and to expect a reasonable number of mistakes, upset feelings, and setbacks. We understand that all of us are wounded and flawed, but that we also are beautiful and worthy of love. We can end our battles with reality and can give ourselves more of what Ellen Burstyn calls "should-less days."

With acceptance comes the possibility of self-forgiveness. As Sharon Salzberg said, "You may search the whole world over and never find a person worthier of love than yourself."

Perhaps the greatest wisdom involves knowing at last how to be good to that crazy baby inside us. When we learn to do that, we can extend mercy to others. We can signal that there is no need for pretense. As we grow, we teach. Our lesson is that it's okay to be the flawed, messed up, contradictory, and marvelous people that we all truly are.

With self-acceptance, we are less likely to be ambitious for recognition or prestige. We may still recognize our competitive nature, but not feel compelled to act upon our competitive impulses. Many of my friends tell me they have less need to impress and achieve. Rather, they feel surges of joy when they empower others.

• • •

WILLOW STOPPED SEEING herself as solely a unit of production. She kept working, but at a different job: caring for Saul. She still had a strong sense of purpose, but she also had times when she was off the clock. She learned that, while it's good to be useful, sometimes it's better not to be useful. She allowed herself to take naps or read the Style section of the *New York Times*. She and Saul told each other more jokes. When she accidentally glanced in a mirror, she was surprised by her own smile. When she heard herself laughing, she thought, "I like this version of me."

In my case, I have perpetually yearned for a bigger life. The quote "Even in Kyoto I yearn for Kyoto" applied to me. But, at seventy, I am more content with my life as it is. Many nights I go to sleep thinking that if this were the last day on earth for me, I would be happy with how I spent it. If I knew I only had one week to live, I don't believe I would change much on my schedule.

Likewise, I have strived much of my life to be a better version of myself. There is a German word, "schlimmbesserung," that means "to be worsened by improvement." Sometimes, I embody that term. My constant quest to be a better person has often kept me from just enjoying my own personality.

Some Buddhists say, "You're perfect the way you are, but you could use a little improvement." That is the way I often feel about myself. To my great relief, I am not always consumed by the desire to be better. Sometimes, I am happy with who I am. I am still a seeker, but I can let myself off the hook for constant self-improvement projects. Sometimes, I accept my quirky personality and my neuroses as part of who I am.

My self-acceptance is a result of a slow-growing process across decades. But every now and then, I'll experience an epiphany that leads to a growth spurt. I allow myself to experience both the cruel and the loving radiance of the universe. I see myself and others clearly, but without judgment. I accept everything.

I experienced such a moment when one June I flew to the Grand Bahama Island with my friend Jan. We had been talking about this trip since we were in our twenties. Neither of our husbands liked beach vacations and, for many years, we couldn't afford such a luxury. But finally, at age sixty-nine, I was ready to go. Jan and I could have fun anywhere—walking on a bike trail or lunching at a hole-in-the-wall café, but now we were on a Caribbean island with its white beaches, blue waves, and stately palms.

Our trip was an elemental experience. We woke with the sunrise and watched the sunset every night. Our schedule was about tides, clouds, light, and flowers. Except for an indoor reading time in the heat of the day, we were outside. We walked on the beach, fixed simple meals, and paddled around in turquoise water. Jan can't swim but I snorkeled and looked at beautiful fish and coral.

At night, I lay on a recliner in the yard and looked at the stars. These stars were liquid and hung low in an unpolluted sky. I could hear the soft cadences of the ocean waves and the breeze in a big coconut palm nearby. One night I peered at the heavens with what I realized was a question. I expected the stars to tell me some great truth. I didn't even know my question, but I trusted the sky would have an answer.

First I experienced the memory of my relatives who had left the world. When I remembered specific moments with most of them, I felt loved and happy. When I recalled the few family members who had caused me great pain, a mask of sorrow swept over my face. My heart hurt as I realized that we never get over things; they stay inside us ready to be remembered and felt.

I looked for a sign—a falling star to tell me that my grandmother was greeting me. I wanted to be recognized in some way by my ancestors or by the stars themselves. After that thought, I had an answer to the question I had not known how to ask.

My answer was simply this: "Let the stars be the stars. That is enough." My busy mind had been poised to immediately concoct expectations, demands, and even stories about what the sky should be doing for me. I had caught myself in the ridiculous position of trying to manipulate the night sky.

"Let the stars be the stars." I felt a wave of peace wash over my body. For that moment, I could simply let things be.

I looked at the sky for a long time. I felt grateful. I sensed the honesty of simply recognizing what is present. In my personal life that could simply mean calling things by their right name. All of my life I had avoided calling pain "pain." I had tried to prettify things, to make them different or better. But what if I could simply call anger "anger"? And call sorrow "sorrow"? What if I could call disloyalty by its true name? What if I could speak the word "bitterness" rather than work so hard to never experience that emotion?

I need not spin anything, deny anything, or claim anything. And yet, I need not stay with any one emotion for a long time. Emotions have a time span and I could merely allow that time span to unfurl. As Leonard Cohen said, "Inner feelings come and go." And when my inner feeling did exit, I could accurately label the emotion that replaced it.

That night I felt I saw the sky from the biggest possible perspective. The stars do not fall up or down. They beam light into our atmosphere. The epiphany on the beach left me calm, joyous, and peaceful. At least for that moment, I felt healed. I also felt that something inside me had changed and that perhaps my life would now be different, more honest and less filled with need.

The great gift of our life stage is authenticity. We have reached a point in our journey when, at least for a moment, we can put down our canoe paddles and look around us. We lose our fears and discover within ourselves a deep well of strength. We can appreciate everything we see. We can be grateful for our own minds, hearts, and bodies. Our maturity and uncrooked heart give us the possibility of seeing our own lives from multiple points of view. We can include all of our ancestors and all living beings in our circle of caring. We can aspire to be kind and present for others. And we can appreciate the constant gifts the world brings us.

CHAPTER 19

The Long View

"The great thing about getting older is that you don't lose all
the other ages you've been." —Madeleine L'Engle

"Live as though your ancestors were living again through you."
—Greek saying

RECENTLY I FOUND my old gold-plated pot for burning incense. Ten years
ago, I had deposited prayers in this pot. They were simple prayers, often
only recorded by a few words, "my sister's behavior," "my brother's health,"
or "my friend's marriage."

I opened this old pot and pulled out all of the prayers. I read them
slowly and tried to remember what events had prompted them. I realized that the prayers had all been answered. Not by anything I did, nor
necessarily by anything that happened to the people I was praying for,
but rather because time had made those particular problems irrelevant.
I was in a different era now. I had new problems. I pondered the blessed
nature of time covering old worries with history. Perhaps this is often
what an answered prayer is, simply a surcease of worry.

As we age, we grow more aware of our place in deep time. We are one drop of water in the flowing river of evolutionary time. Our life histories reach back to the beginning of the universe and our hominid lineage is fifteen to twenty million years old. We are connected to ancient and majestic rhythms and cycles and we are here now, sharing this moment in time with our friends and family, our country, seven billion other people, and all living beings. This sense for deep time and interconnection often comes to us late in life. When we deeply experience it, we feel both a profound sorrow and a deep joy.

Time is a great teacher of perspective. If we allow ourselves to be present and if we work to understand our experiences, the tincture of time can heal us. Our capacity to make mistakes is endless and suffering in its many forms is always with us. Yet over the course of our lives we learn that humans are wired to absorb adverse shocks. This develops in us a certain respect for resilience and the indefatigable nature of hope. Looking back on our own lives, we can see an endless cycle of crisis and growth.

"By the time we're sixty-five years old, we've experienced a lot of stuff," my cousin Steve said. No doubt about that. When we look back, we find joy and sorrow, mistakes and victories, moments on golden rivers, and nights lost in the dark. We can see ourselves from babyhood on.

I can barely identify with the woman I was at twenty-one when I sold my blood to buy a retro black flapper dress covered in dangling, sparkling black beads. When I walked in it, I shimmered like a slender black flame. I can hardly imagine the young woman who bought that dress. Now, I would only sell my blood for a matter of life or death. I mostly wear sweatpants and T-shirts and the last thing I want to do is attract attention.

Yet, if we look for continuities, we can find them. I most enjoy now what I most enjoyed at age ten. I like reading, studying, swimming, walking, and being with my friends and family. No matter what life stage I've been in, I've liked to take care of people and animals. Recently, I spoke with my best friend from eighth grade, who recalled that I often suggested that we lie in the grass and look at the sky. I still do that with my family and friends.

When I was a young girl, I read for hours a day. When I was young, I read *A Tree Grows in Brooklyn*, *The Diary of Anne Frank*, and *To Kill a Mockingbird*. I loved biographies of women such as Helen Keller, Madame Curie, and Eleanor Roosevelt. This reading acquainted me with our human capacities for good and ill. I still spend my time reading books that help me understand our complicated, multifaceted human experience across time and place.

I reflect upon the events of my life, which began less than a year after the end of WWII. Our generation was shaped by the Korean conflict; the Cold War; the Cuban Revolution; the civil rights movement; the assassinations of John F. Kennedy, Martin Luther King Jr., and Bobby Kennedy; the Vietnam War; the impact of climate change, 9/11; and the wars in the Middle East.

My life was also shaped by people I met along the way, such as the Swedish immigrant woman who taught me to make pottery, an excellent high school English teacher, my anthropology professors at the University of California at Berkeley, certain professors from my graduate program in clinical psychology, and my long-term advisers and friends from publishing. Since 1972, I've been in a community of local friends and we have shaped each other's tastes, values, and attitudes.

However, my most important influences have been family. I can see across six generations of time, and, before I die, if I am very lucky, I will see seven. This long view of family helps me reflect upon questions such as "What is temperament?" "What are the effects of parenting? Of culture?" "What is in the blood?" "How did I come to be who I am today?"

When I was a girl these questions were easier to parse. We all had more or less the same culture and opportunities in Beaver City, Nebraska.

We were exposed to the same news of the world. This gave us an advantage in sorting out what were cultural, familial, and individual characteristics. I am glad I had a small-town childhood. Today we often do not know the extended kin of the people around us.

My two families of origin were very different from each other. My dad's family was Irish. They were informal, physically affectionate, and gregarious. My mother's family from Scotland was puritanical and formal. They emphasized the importance of education, moral responsibility, and civic duty. I am a mixture of the two sets of kin.

My mother and maternal grandmother most influenced my values. Grandmother Page felt her duty was to raise me to be a deeply moral person. Our conversations were about books we had read and the choices that I made about friends and activities. She encouraged me to think about how I could be of use to the world. She called me "My Mary."

My sense of duty came from this grandmother. She taught me to think only of others. Perhaps I learned that lesson a little too well! I have worked this last decade of my life to learn to think more about my own needs and joys.

My mother was the only doctor in our county and she did the school physicals, the autopsies, the deliveries, the surgeries, and the medical emergencies on the highway and at the racetrack. She didn't tolerate fools gladly. She couldn't stand hypochondriacs, slackers, or complainers. She herself was always on the go and she expected us children to keep moving too.

She was a good mother, but she wasn't around much and she had little tolerance for our emotional needs. If we asked to stay home from school because we were sick, she would say, "That's fine. Let me give you a big penicillin shot first and you'll have to be in your bed all day with only tea." That attitude discouraged malingering. Sadly, it also discouraged much honest expression of pain.

Across the years, we also may learn from certain people how we do not want to be. The miserly uncle, the cruel teacher, or the harsh parent can inspire us to develop in a different direction. Many a woman has shaped herself by deciding that she will be the opposite of a powerful negative example. One friend of mine with an alcoholic and neglectful mother told me, "When I became a mother, I vowed to give my children a different kind of parenting. I didn't drink or smoke. I baked cookies and led a Girl Scout troop. I never missed any of my kids' events and I listened to them. I knew who they were."

Fate and choice intertwine to create the person we are. We can clearly see the role luck and chance play. For example, Jim happened to be in my class in graduate school. I asked him to be my study buddy and later we chose to date. Had I not started graduate school in a particular place and time, I would not have lived this particular life. We all have many stories like this.

From our vantage point, we can see our lives as braided rivers with many strands coming together and interweaving. We can see the gentle turns and the oxbows, the ice jams, and the spring flows. We can begin to understand what is the riverbed and what is the river, or what is long-lasting and what is ephemeral.

This view affords us inspiration, joy, solace, and practical advice. Examining our pasts add depths to relationships, helps us understand ourselves, and allows us to feel deeply connected with people from our past and present times and the future, long after we are gone.

At our age, we can solve many problems simply because we've encountered them before and learned how to proceed. When someone shares her anguish with us, we know how to listen and comfort her. We know how to entertain or soothe a child. We can plan a wedding or a funeral and behave well when we are in emotional or physical pain. We can identify the catastrophes that deepened our hearts and the people and events that changed the way we looked at the world and enlarged our moral imaginations.

• • •

AUBURN-HAIRED WILLOW OFTEN reflected on the long view. Many members of her family had been killed in the Holocaust. When she looked at the few pictures she had of her grandparents and relatives, she thought about how different her life would have been without the war and genocide. Her parents would have stayed in Russia, closely connected to the town where their families had lived for hundreds of years. Instead, they lived in New York City and Willow had grown up speaking English.

When Willow pictured her childhood, she saw her parents dusting cigar cases or counting out the take at the end of the day. She smelled her mother's borscht or sweet and sour cabbage. She remembered her college years or her graduation speech. She thought of her classmates, many of whom were still in touch. She recalled one teacher, a French woman who taught social work, who inspired her idealism and helped her understand the concept of professional ethics.

Willow was deeply grateful she met Saul, who had been a constant good person in her life. She regretted that she had been a busy and inattentive wife for most of their marriage. But now, she was making up for lost time. She felt their marriage was stronger and better than ever. Living with Parkinson's disease had made them both more carefree, and more grateful. She felt honored to have shared her life with Saul.

Still, Willow's greatest pride came from her professional life. She felt happy when she remembered times she had helped clients find a home, a doctor, or a job. She relished her memories of Ruby, Myron, and many other clients. She recalled her favorite staff and the women she had mentored. She remembered the holiday parties when she bought pizza and apple cider and everyone danced to Cuban music.

She knew she had steered her agency through hard times and made a big difference in the lives of the chronically mentally ill in New York City. "My mother and father would be proud of me," she thought. "I've done what I could to make my piece of the planet a better place."

• • •

IN AUSTIN, SYLVIA looks back on her life with a mixture of sadness and pride. Her parents were sharecroppers who never had much of anything to enjoy. She was the one to make good grades and bump herself into the middle class. She wishes her parents could have enjoyed some of Lewis's and her pleasures. They'd taken a trip with Lenore to Padre Island on the Gulf of Mexico, and they'd driven to New Orleans one year for Mardi Gras. Together, they'd savored good food, country music, and the kindness of their neighbors and church members.

Sylvia's deepest regrets are about Lenore. Lenore had been a lovely, bright-spirited child who'd seemed destined for happiness. Sylvia has all of her little sports trophies, writing, and artwork. However, remembering Lenore now is complicated. Sylvia's heart hurts when she thinks of her daughter. She feels a mix of emotions about Lenore—anger, fear, sorrow, and fierce maternal love.

Sylvia is grateful that she and Lewis have the grandchildren. They give them joy, a connection to Lenore, and a mission. She takes pride in the ways she and Lewis are parenting. She's saving a few dollars a week so that someday they can all take a vacation. She hopes they can live long enough to raise Max and Gracie. And, at night when she can't sleep, Sylvia says prayers for Lenore. If Lenore ever comes home, they will take her in. She is family and "family" is a sacred word to Sylvia.

• • •

WHEN REDHEADED EMMA is lonely and sad, she has a strategy that relies on decades of memories. All of her life, when she had been in beautiful places, she would think, "I am going to bottle this moment and take it with me." Now, when times get tough, she can pull out that bottle and take a big sip of Yellowstone or the Pacific Ocean.

• • •

OUR LONG HISTORIES with friends and family allow us to give them the love they most need in the present. I remember my husband as a twenty-two-year-old long-haired musician singing "Teach Your Children" and "The Green, Green Grass of Home." I can see him as the father of a newborn, the director of a mental health clinic next to a chicken hatchery, and a marathon runner. I can envision all of Jim's life stages in the gray-haired man who does crossword puzzles in our living room. We've shared forty-five years together and I know what makes him happy, angry, or sad. Because I know all that, I can make him laugh or comfort him when he is low.

My brother told a story about a tailor who wanted to visit the new pope. His small parish took up a collection to send him to Rome. The pope was touched by the story of the small parish and this man's long journey. He gave the tailor a personal audience and they talked for a considerable time. When the man returned to his town, the parish had a party for him and asked him about the new pope. He had only one thing to say: "The pope wears a size forty-four medium."

We don't see the world as it is, but rather as we are. If we are angry and bitter, we find proof of hostility wherever we look. If we are trusting, we look for evidence of kindness. Growth requires us to constantly expand our points of view. We began as an infant with ourselves as the only relevant person. Later, if we develop properly, we appreciate the views of our families and our school friends. As adults, we can continue to expand our capacities for empathy with all the people we meet. If we are curious, we don't just look for evidence that confirms our narrowest opinions, but rather we try to understand more about everyone and everything. We yearn to see the world through the broadest of all lenses. By taking the longest possible view, we can experience gratitude, wisdom, and a sense for the moral continuity of our lives. This strengthens our identities and brings us peace and connection.

Time and moral imagination are the great healers of the human psyche. One summer afternoon I attended a naming ceremony for a one-year-old girl born in Nebraska to Mohamed and Tambu from Sierra Leone. I was Isatu's honorary grandmother whose role it was to offer a blessing. People had come from four states to meet in a community garden outside of town. Mohamed played African music. His kinsmen killed a small goat in a ritualized and gentle way, then divided up the meat for all of the guests. Isatu played with the other children under the trees in her satiny white dress.

As I was leaving, Mohamed brought me a kola nut and explained that they are part of every ceremony in his village. Kola nuts represent life, respect, and significance. The nut is about the size of a chestnut and reddish brown. He said that at first I wouldn't like the taste, but to keep chewing. They are bitter when first tasted, but then, with chewing, they become sweeter and, after a while, the mouth feels clean, all bitterness gone. He said that the kola nut teaches a lesson—many things that are not sweet become that way with patience and perseverance. I bit into the nut and felt the urge to spit it out immediately. But Mohamed was right. As I chewed, the bitterness disappeared and my mouth felt refreshed. I doubt I'll be eating many kola nuts in my future, but I'd like to remember the lesson. Time can take the sting out of life and make it sweeter.

If we are growing, we experience our circle of caring expand into a profound sense of connection to all living beings. We feel a radical empathy. There is no "us" and no "them." In our hearts, we are all the same. My friend Lynne describes this as "deep happiness." She can look around at almost any gathering and feel an upwelling of gratitude for the people she is with. When she hikes in wilderness areas, she's continually amazed by all of the beauty and wonder. "I have learned to let a lot of things go," Lynne said. "I am sometimes able to accept uncertainty as a gift rather than something to be afraid of."

With time, many of us become more forgiving and more capable of love. We can look back tenderly to the times when we were young and vulnerable to forces that no longer crash around us. We can love those lost girls and nurture the lonely, vulnerable, and scared girl that is still inside us. And, we can turn that love outward toward all living beings.

CHAPTER 20

Everything Is Illuminated

"We live in the womb of the universe and everything is designed to help us be safe, happy, and loved. We only must choose to notice this beauty all around us." —Joanne Friday

"Old age is not an illness, it is a timeless ascent. As power diminishes, we grow toward more light." —May Sarton

EMMA PLANNED A family reunion at a mountain cabin by a lake to celebrate Chris's seventieth birthday. She packed peaches and cherries, bread and cheese, and homemade energy bars. She baked Chris a lemon sheet cake and bought seventy candles. Along with her trepidation and hope, she loaded up the board games, lawn chairs, and sunscreen. With her kids and their children in the same place for forty-eight hours, there were bound to be some meltdowns and arguments. Sure enough, there were.

One of the twins wandered off and everyone stressed out looking for her. Alice and Emma's oldest son's wife had an argument that started with a discussion about whether it was safe to use mayonnaise on sand-wiches packed for a day hike, but escalated into a metaphorical discussion of who was the better homemaker. While the women were arguing about who purchased the most organic produce, Emma slipped out the door.

She walked about a block from the cabin and lay down on the soft forest floor under some aspen. That contact with the earth always grounded her emotionally. As she watched the clouds float over the snow-capped peaks to the north, she breathed deeply. She breathed in calm-ness and breathed out stress. By the time she stood up, she was centered and ready to rejoin the party.

Sunday afternoon everyone gathered under sunny skies. The youngest children played by the water and the teenagers tried to catch trout. The adults sat in lawn chairs, drinking beer and laughing at each other's jokes. Chris got his shoes and pants wet untangling a fishing line. More laughter ensued.

Emma sat a little to the side and savored this good family moment. Her oldest son passed out popcorn and paper cups of chardonnay. The children constructed towers on the shore. The unsuccessful but happy trout fishers cast back into the blue water. Even the two women who had been fighting had their heads together and were smiling. She remem-bered a line from a Frost poem she had learned in high school. "Earth's the right place for love: I don't know where it's likely to go better."

All of a sudden, Emma felt the ions in the air change and she was totally immersed in the moment. She felt as if she were in the heart of the universe. She experienced a great physical rush of pure happiness. Time stopped entirely and all the voices around her faded. The entire atmosphere shimmered with what Emma could only describe as bliss.

• • •

BLISS, ILLUMINATION, AWE, and wonder all signify experiences that are hard to describe with ordinary language. In fact, they can only be described metaphorically. Indeed, in a state of awe everything becomes a metaphor.

Bliss, like orgasm, comes easier after our first experience. After that, we know we can make it happen again. Moments of bliss can occur all across our life spans, and, as we age, such moments may become daily occurrences. When I was a mother of young children and working full-time, I rarely slowed down for bliss. Usually I was tired, rushed, and preoccupied with duties and chores. Now, with a more relaxed life, I can move slowly enough to appreciate what is happening all around me.

Awe gives us a different sense of ourselves. We feel smaller, humbler, and more connected to all others. We don't feel entitled or narcissistic, but rather part of a common humanity.

Some people are predisposed to awe. I know a few women who wander around ecstatic. And, Emily Dickinson wrote, "Life is so astonishing that it leaves very little time for anything else."

For others, bliss is hard-won. For many years, Sylvia had no energy for bliss. Her life was filled with work and stress. Then, one night something miraculous happened.

It was an ordinary weeknight. Sylvia called everyone to dinner. Lewis insisted Max put on a shirt before coming to the table and that made Max so angry that he threw his plate of lasagna on the floor. Lewis left the table immediately and went into the den to watch TV. Gracie started to cry. Sylvia put Gracie's dinner on a tray and set her down by Lewis. Then she held Max in a tight embrace until he settled down. She finished her own plate of lasagna and cleaned up the mess.

Later, she went up to tuck Max in. They read a chapter of *Little House on the Prairie*, then knelt by the bed and said their prayers. They both prayed for Lenore and for a better day tomorrow. When Sylvia kissed

Max good night, he touched her cheek and said, "Grandma, you are so beautiful."

Sylvia looked in his eyes and realized that he meant it. She was old, fat, and crippled, but Max thought she was beautiful. She felt a warmth enfold her. Max looked as if he were made of light. She was exactly where she most wanted to be. She knew she would never have a better moment. This one was perfect.

• • •

ALL OF KESTREL's life, her main emotion had been worry. She had been hyper-vigilant, always monitoring others for signs they might hurt her in some way. But, this last year, Evelyn's cancer and death, the family reunion, and Becca's kindness had changed her. For the first time in her life, she felt relaxed. That was such a new emotional state that it took her a few months to even recognize and label it.

Back in Seattle, Becca was a regular part of her life. Together, they attended Pride events, worked out, and fixed evenings meals. While Becca checked over student papers, Kestrel did crosswords. Kestrel knew Becca's family and mother. She was even going to the family Christmas at Becca's mother's house.

One warm day early in December, Becca called and invited her to drive down to Ruby Beach. On the drive down, they talked about what to take to Christmas dinner and their plans for an alcohol-free New Year's Eve party at Becca's place. They arrived at noon and after sharing a rotisserie chicken and some pears, they walked along the beach holding hands and looking at the beautiful rocks.

Kestrel could hear the soft breaking of the waves and the wind in the Douglas firs and redwoods. She could smell the salty moist air. They ambled along the shore looking at rocks most of the afternoon. Around sunset, they found a silver piece of driftwood and sat down to watch the waves.

Kestrel took Becca's hand and did not let go. When Becca and she held hands, Kestrel's breathing slowed and deepened. Suddenly, she saw Becca as someone like her, struggling to find herself, wanting to be good and to feel loved. With that realization, her protective wall fell away from her just as old bark falls from trees. She felt as if she could trust not only Becca but other people too. She wasn't afraid.

She melted into a peacefulness that had never been part of her experience. Before she was even aware she was speaking, she said, "I love you."

Both women began to cry.

• • •

MANY OF US discover ways to experience bliss and awe when we are most in pain. Our losses and sorrows propel us toward that which is redemptive. We must find an emotional state to balance our despair. Great personal suffering can sometimes deepen our souls to the point they crack open and let in great beauty.

When our hearts crack open, we feel an identification and empathy with all who have suffered. We pray for not only ourselves but for everyone who has suffered. At last we have joined the community of grief and loss, rage and fear. We do not feel alone in our pain, but rather deeply connected to all those who have felt pain. This experience induces wonder.

Saul and Willow were exhausted when they returned home from Saul's monthly Parkinson's assessment. They had been stuck in crosstown traffic for over an hour. The cabdriver kept talking and cursing, and horns and sirens frayed their tattered nerves. Saul's doctor had told them that Saul was losing strength and muscle control. He advised Saul to eat only pureed foods as the muscles in his throat were weakening and he could easily choke on a piece of steak or apple. Both Saul and Willow had winced at the word "pureed."

Their beautiful and quiet apartment was a relief. Saul sat down in the one chair he could still get in and out of. It faced west so that he could see the sunset, but tonight, it was raining hard.

That night during dinner Saul choked on a small piece of mashed potato. His face turned crimson and he signaled to Willow that he needed the Heimlich maneuver. The doctor had shown her how to do it and had given her a handout, but Willow couldn't recall how it worked or remember where her written instructions were. Meanwhile, Saul kept choking.

Willow was terrified and furious with herself for not knowing what to do. But, she ran behind Saul, grabbed him just below his ribs and jerked as hard as she could. A bit of food flew out of his mouth and across the table onto her chair. Saul was still choking, but he took a breath and then another. Both of them began to sob. It had been so close. Neither of them had ever been that scared before.

After they quit crying, they no longer wanted any dinner. They just stared at each other across their almost-full plates. After a few minutes, Willow cleared the table and helped Saul into the living room. She lit some tall white candles and put on some Ravel. The rain continued to fall in big splats. However, the beautiful music and the candlelight afforded them some kind of peace.

Saul took her hand and said, "When I was choking, I was scared because I couldn't breathe, but I'm not afraid of dying. I've had a great life with you. When God hits the stop button, I will be ready."

Willow looked at his wise and kind face. He was such a gentleman, so erudite and eager to please her. She said, "I wouldn't have missed a minute of the life we had together. L'Chaim."

• • •

BLISS IS AN illuminating experience followed by a great feeling of acceptance and calmness. Joy and gratitude are part of this experience. We hold at the same time the deepest sorrow of the world and most exalted happiness. We experience the double nature of reality. After the destruction by terrorists of the promenade in Nice, France, my friend Jan said, "What a world we live in, so beautiful and so bleak."

Bliss feels both utterly different from ordinary reality and more real. It is as if the scales have fallen from our eyes and we can see clearly. Our defensiveness, vanities, and problems all vanish in the context of a bigger, purer reality. The beauty that we miss in our ordinary consciousness sparkles all around us. We are pelted by epiphanies and gobsmacked by awe.

Not everyone experiences bliss as they age, but it is never too late to look for it. And, if we look for it, we will find it, as Dr. Zhivago taught me so long ago. If we make good choices and have skillful intentions, we will be primed for bliss and joy. As one of my friends put it, "When I was younger I felt bliss when I had sex or ran a marathon, but now I can feel it looking at the tomatoes at a farmers market."

One of the quickest pathways to bliss is to experience a life-threatening illness. All of a sudden life's sweetness and tragedy unfurl before us. When we hear that we may only have a short time to live, life seems incredibly precious.

My friend Jackie is near the end of her battle with clear cell cancer. Nine months ago, when she received her diagnosis, she was the vibrant director of a statewide organization. She couldn't believe her bad luck. She had lived a healthy lifestyle and had never missed a day of work because of illness. At first, Jackie kept working at her office, then for a short while she worked from home. But now she is too weak from her chemotherapy and radiation treatments to continue.

Shortly after Jackie's diagnosis, her only child became engaged to her boyfriend of several years. When Jackie was between treatments, the family celebrated the wedding. For that one day, Jackie became a healthy woman. She carried in chairs, welcomed everyone at the door, stood by her daughter during the service, sang and danced with her relatives, and, afterward, helped with the dishes. I was not surprised by Jackie's behavior. No matter what, that is how she would behave at her daughter's wedding.

In early September, Jackie came over to sit by the lake. As she slowly walked to a bench, I observed how thin and fragile she had become. She said that her bones were breaking because of the cancer. She regularly took pain pills although she didn't like them. She knew she was supposed to eat, but food made her sick.

We sat in the late-afternoon sun and looked west through backlit prairie grasses. The cottonwoods' gold and green leaves rustled above us. A few feet away, fishermen cast their lines and kayaks slid by us.

As we sat and watched the bucolic scene, she told me that she had experienced all the stages of grief. At first, she was outraged. She was only in her fifties, and she wanted to work for another twenty years. She was also angry because her daughter would be left behind with no parents. Jackie questioned why an evildoer or someone who wanted to die could not die instead of her.

Jackie loved being alive, but the constant chemo and radiation treatments had taken their toll. She was trying punishing experimental treatments that exhausted her and left her confused. Her emotions were hard to control, but she continued to frame her life in the most positive ways that she could. For example, her daughter had taken a leave of absence for the last few months. She told me that this cancer meant she was probably spending more time with her daughter than she would ever have had she stayed well.

During this time, Jackie experienced both bliss and heartache. She was sick and facing death but her ability to receive and give love had greatly increased, as had her capacity for gratitude. Until she had cancer, Jackie had never realized how many people deeply loved her. She'd been an independent woman, almost phobic about accepting people's care. But her illness taught her to welcome offers of help. She often found herself weeping with gratitude for the kindness she received.

As Jackie and I watched the grasses backlit by sunlight, and the clouds reflected on the lake, she searched for enchantment. She needed it. The swallows dive-bombed around us and a meadowlark on a fence post sang us her beautiful song. Jackie breathed deeply and swept her arm across the landscape. She recited her favorite lines from Willa Cather, "This is happiness—to be dissolved into something complete and great."

None of us know when we will die. The implications, though, are the same for all of us. We want to make each day as revelatory as we possibly can. We can all orchestrate bliss. Retreat centers and other places designed to help people heal from addiction or traumas are often situated in calm, beautiful places. It is this very beauty that becomes the agent of healing.

Illumination often comes from small experiences that grow by attention. Illumination leads to more illumination. We can achieve it strolling through a park looking at red maples burnished by light, when worshiping in church, praying or meditating in our bedrooms, or laughing with a friend. We can experience it looking into the face of a loved one. These things, if carefully attended, can feel like redemption.

In Nebraska one guaranteed way to experience this bliss is to visit the Sandhill cranes during their great migration stay along the Platte River in March. As many as 500,000 cranes wheel onto the river as the sun sets, and the sky sings with their calls, a sound you feel you heard before you were born.

Every spring I celebrate by visiting Rowe Sanctuary and spending the evening in a blind along the Platte. The cranes land just after dusk and form islands in the silver river. The sky is filled with birds. Their calls blot out all other sounds. It seems as if the world were made of cranes.

Every year I experience the best crane year ever. That is because every year I feel wonder and we can't parse wonder. Present wonder seems the best only because it is happening at the moment.

We have a three-legged cat that comes onto our property to eat the food that we set out for birds and foxes. The first time my grandson saw this cat, he burst into tears. She is skinny, mangy, and most likely perpetually hungry. She can't run very fast and could easily be the victim of an owl, hawk, or coyote. Yet, somehow, she has survived for the last couple of years.

This winter, after a cold, gray week, the temperature rose by thirty degrees and the sun came out. I looked out my window and saw the three-legged cat eating birdseed on our driveway. After her feast, she rolled around on her back with her paws in the air. Then she licked herself and stretched, clearly blissed out to be lying in a sunbeam. I thought to myself, "I want to feel as ecstatic as that cat."

Bliss doesn't happen because we are perfect or problem-free but rather because over the years we have become wise enough to occasionally be present for the moment. We have acquired the capacity to appreciate what simply is. This state is both the simplest and the most complex of human experiences. Yet, in spite of our situations, whatever they are, we all can have our days when we feel like a three-legged cat drenched in sunlight.

All great truths are paradoxes. We are all both together and alone. Time is everything and nothing. Life is joyous and life is tragic. The Cape of Good Hope and the Cape of Storms are literally and figuratively the same place. In a state of bliss, all paradoxes can be held without tension. Cause and effect may exist, but it is hard to tell which is which. Everything seems so connected and inevitable.

Dear sisters, I hope that we can experience bliss. I want us to sense how big life is—how intense, joyful, painful, complicated, and beautiful our lives can be. Let us embrace everything. This can be our rescue as we navigate this last stretch of the river with its treacherous currents, quicksand, deep clear waters, and silver sunsets.

ACKNOWLEDGMENTS

As with any book about the human experience, I'm tempted to thank everyone I've met in my entire life. All of my interactions have greatly influenced my views of what humans do for each other and to each other. Please, everyone who I have ever met, consider yourself thanked. You have all been my teachers.

Specifically, I would like to thank the people I interviewed—Eloise Kloefkorn, Sally Herrin, Cynthia Hischke, Pat Leach, Kay Young, Marge Manglitz, Paul Olson, Jan Enstrom and Scott Svoboda, Nan Schweiger, Jeanine Bray, Carmen Grant, Gretchen and Ardie Davis, Barbara di Bernard, Judith Gibson, Renee Sans Souci, Diane "Jeep" Ries, Diana Lofredo, Holly Kaye, Lynne Iser, Rondi Lightmark, Mary Lou Mittan, Rich Simon, Regina Edington, Florine Joseph, and Paula D. Washington.

I would like to thank my readers and assistants—Natalie O'Neal, Jan Zegers, Aubrey Streit Krug, Mary Dickinson, Kim Hachiya, Jamie Pipher, Sara Gilliam, Laura Wertz, and Jane Isay. Kudos to John Gilliam, my technology consultant, who kept me writing in spite of my damaged hands and lack of computer savvy and to Larry Williams of the Malone Center, Carmen Grant and Christy Hargesheimer, my scouts. Thanks also to my consultant on hospice, Jeanine Bray.

Many thanks to my agent and river guide of thirty years, Susan Lee Cohen, my wonderful editor, Nancy Miller, and to the team at Bloomsbury Publishing who believed in me and helped me launch this boat.

Bless the Prairie Trout, my writers group since the 1980s, who have been with me every mile of my river journey.

And finally, thanks to my family, my husband, Jim, my son, Zeke, my daughter, Sara, my son-in-law, John, my daughter-in-law, Jamie, and the five grands—Kate, Aidan, Claire, Coltrane, and Otis. Words cannot touch my gratitude to them. They hold my life in place.

INDEX

life partners
  and balance, 187–88
  caregiving for, 60–61, 66–67, 68, 73–74,
    78–80, 113–14, 149, 227
  changes in, 184–86, 188
  and commitment, 186, 191, 192, 193
  and conflicts, 184, 185, 187, 189, 194
  and divorce, 104–6, 148, 178–80, 187,
    190–91, 192
  and emotional and social space, 186–87
  and expectations, 190
  loss of, 6, 22–23, 82
  and outside friendships, 186–87
  and pain, 188–89
  and same-sex marriage, 190, 191–92
life span, length of, 3, 186
life stages. *See also* adolescence; middle age to
  old age transition
  challenges of, 18–19, 84
  joy in, 232–33
  and memories, 238
lifetimes within a lifetime, continuities and
  discontinuities of, 14–15, 19, 25, 29–30,
  240
Lindberg, Henrik, 84
loneliness
  challenges of, 10, 83–84
  coping with, 94–95
  and cultivation of relationships,
    88, 90–91
  and grief, 74, 75
  and health issues, 84, 90–91
  and other people's decisions, 85–88
  and scars from childhood traumas,
    88–90
  and sexuality, 38
  solitude compared to, 84, 91–92, 95
lookism, 10
loss. *See also* grief
  coping with, 3, 4, 6, 8, 10, 18
  of life partners, 6, 22–23, 82

  and loneliness, 84, 86
  old age accompanied by, 7
Lyubomirsky, Sonja, 111

Macy, Joanna, 24
Malone Center, 141–43
Marie Antoinette, Queen of France, 207
maximizers, of expectations, 129
Mead, Margaret, 16, 30
meaning
  and building a good day, 123
  and caregiving, 62
  constructing narratives with, 16, 148, 149,
    159
  exploration of, 19
  and grief, 82
  skills of building, 6
Means, Russell, 145
Media Diversity and Social Change
  Initiative, 27
meditation, 65, 103, 179, 221, 226, 249
memories
  and building a good day, 134
  and changes in narratives, 148
  and grandchildren, 208
  integrated memories, 41
  and narratives, 41, 148, 149, 150, 152,
    153–56, 158–59, 238
  and relationships, 183
  sensory memories, 153–54
  and solitude, 91
men, roles of, 16
middle age to old age transition
  adaptations in, 3, 19, 22
  as "both/and" experience, 8, 20
  and chronological age, 3
  contradictions of, 20
  cultural challenges of, 18
  developmental perspective on, 17
  and identity, 3, 4, 17
  journey through, 7